KT-478-764

Understanding
Pregnancy

Dr Norman C. Smith

Published by Family Doctor Publications Limited
in association with the British Medical Association

© Family Doctor Publications 2005–2006
Updated 2006

Family Doctor Publications, PO Box 4664, Poole, Dorset BH15 1NN

ISBN-10: 1-903474-515
ISBN-13: 978-1903474-518

Contents

About the author

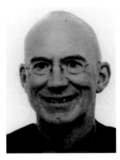

Dr Norman C. Smith has been Consultant Obstetrician with subspecialty expertise in fetal and maternal medicine at Aberdeen Maternity Hospital since 1986. He is a medical graduate from Aberdeen University, training in Aberdeen, Cape Town and Glasgow. He has written extensively on various aspects of pregnancy.

Planning a pregnancy

Prepare yourself

If you are planning a pregnancy, you may find some or all of the answers to any concerns that you may have in this book. If you think that you require specific information and advice, you may need pre-pregnancy counselling from a professional health worker. You should certainly have specialised advice if you have a medical condition such as diabetes or a family history of a genetic disorder, such as the blood condition sickle-cell disease.

It is better to plan to have a baby rather than find yourself pregnant by chance. This is because you can prepare your body so that it is in an ideal physical state to carry the pregnancy. You can have a positive mental attitude and look forward to what is going to happen. Such preparation will give your developing baby the best chance in life. However, we know that almost half of all pregnancies are unplanned.

General health measures
Your weight

Do you know your weight and more importantly what it should be? Charts have been calculated to show the ideal body weight for a given height. These charts calculate what is termed your 'body mass index' (BMI) and show the range of weight that is considered to be healthy for your height. If you check your BMI on the chart on page 3, you may find that you are too heavy or too light for your height. Obviously, it is best to be in the healthy zone. If you are overweight, you are more likely to have pregnancy complications and more likely to have a heavy baby which may make your delivery more difficult. If you are very underweight, you are more likely to have a light baby who may show signs of being underfed before birth.

Your diet

Take care with your diet and try to eat healthy foods that you enjoy. This is not difficult to do with the wide variety of options in the food stores today. You don't need to spend money in health and specialist food shops to achieve a healthy balanced diet.

There are four main food groups required for a balanced diet:

1. Starchy foods (bread, potatoes, pasta)

2. Fruit and vegetables

3. Meat, fish, eggs, nuts and pulses

4. Dairy products.

You should try to eat something from each of these food groups every day. This will give you most of the minerals and vitamins that you need for a good start to your pregnancy.

What should you weigh?

- The body mass index (BMI) is a useful measure of healthy weight
- Find out your height in metres and weight in kilograms
- Calculate your BMI like this

$$BMI = \frac{\text{Your weight (kg)}}{[\text{Your height (metres)} \times \text{Your height (metres)}]}$$

$$\text{e.g. } 24.8 = \frac{70}{[1.68 \times 1.68]}$$

- You are recommended to try to maintain a BMI in the range 20–25
- The chart below is an easier way of estimating your BMI. Read off your height and your weight. The point where the lines cross in the chart indicates your BMI

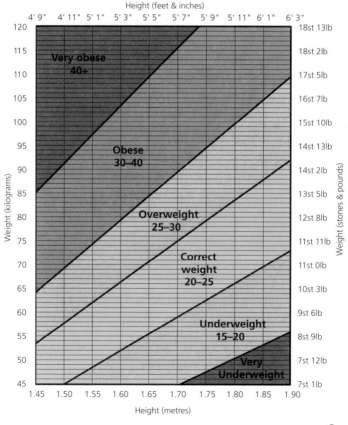

The only vitamin that you need to add to your diet is folic acid, which is a preventive treatment. Taken before pregnancy and for the early weeks of pregnancy it will greatly reduce the chances of your baby having a birth defect called spina bifida (see page 13). You can buy folic acid at most pharmacies without a prescription. You should take 400 micrograms every day, starting three months before you want to fall

Balancing your diet

During pregnancy, you need to eat a healthy diet to ensure that your developing baby obtains enough essential nutrients. You should aim to balance your intake of the different food groups into the following approximate proportions.

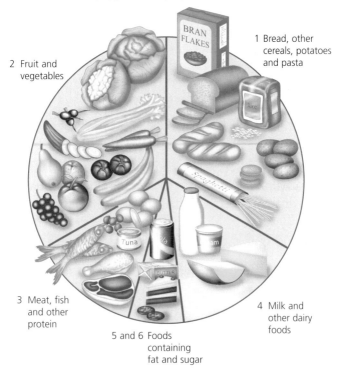

2 Fruit and vegetables

1 Bread, other cereals, potatoes and pasta

3 Meat, fish and other protein

5 and 6 Foods containing fat and sugar

4 Milk and other dairy foods

A balanced diet

Foods should be included in your diet in the following relative proportions. However, you do not need to measure quantities of food very accurately except on medical advice.

Food group	Daily serving
1. Starchy foods: bread, rice, pasta, cereals, potatoes, sweet potatoes	Four or more portions per day. Use this food group to satisfy your appetite
2. Fruit and vegetables: fresh, frozen, dried or liquefied, including leafy green vegetables	At least five portions per day
3. Meat, fish, eggs, nuts and pulses: pulses include lentils, kidney beans and other types of beans without sugary sauces	Two portions per day
4. Dairy products: including milk, yoghurt, hard cheeses, fromage frais	Three portions per day
5. Spreading and cooking fats	In small amounts
6. Sugar and confectionery	Eat only limited quantities and do not eat instead of nutrient-dense foods (that is, those in the first four groups)

Foods to avoid during pregnancy

Certain foods can affect the health and development of your growing baby.

- **Liver, liver pâtés, fish liver oil capsules**
  In excess these give you too much vitamin A which has been associated with birth defects such as bone deformities.

- **Certain soft cheeses**
  Soft cheese, for example brie, camembert, goats' cheese, and blue-vein cheeses, for example Danish blue, Stilton may carry the bacterium *Listeria* which can cause you a harmless bout of diarrhoea, although sometimes it can lead to a miscarriage.

- **Chilled or undercooked meats and unpasteurised milk (cows' or goats') or cheeses**
  These may cause a flu-like illness resulting from *Toxoplasma*, a small parasite that affects cats and which can damage the eyes of the fetus or cause a miscarriage.

- **Undercooked eggs and raw egg products**
  Products such as home-made mayonnaise or chocolate mousse may cause salmonella poisoning which can result in severe diarrhoea and may lead to a miscarriage.

- **Peanuts**
  Peanuts can affect you, especially if you, your partner or close relatives have a history of severe allergies. When a mother-to-be eats peanuts in pregnancy there seems to be an increased risk that the baby will become allergic to peanuts in childhood.

pregnant and continue to take it until 12 weeks after your last period. Folic acid is a B vitamin and is necessary for normal growth and development of the whole pregnancy.

Clearly if your pregnancy was unplanned you will not be able to take a protective dose of folic acid before conception. Start taking it as soon as you suspect that you might be pregnant; even without folic acid protection, the risk of a serious birth defect is still small – around one in 200 babies.

If you suffer from epilepsy or have had a previous pregnancy affected by spina bifida, your developing baby has a greater risk of spina bifida. You should take a higher dose of folic acid (five milligrams or 5 mg), and you will need a prescription for this from your doctor. If you are a vegetarian and do not eat any dairy products (a vegan) you will also need to take a vitamin B_{12} supplement.

Finally on the subject of diet, you should recognise that most of us eat too much sugar, which will in time increase weight. Your developing baby will also become too heavy if you eat too much. Sugar is present in excessive amounts in chocolate bars, sweet fizzy drinks, sauces and many other processed foods. You should reduce your consumption of foods that are high in sugar or, better still, stop eating them altogether. The general health message is that the pleasure of eating sugar (and fat in crisps, chips, sausages, etc.) leads to poor health. Pregnancy is a good time to reduce the amount that you eat of these foods.

Eating the foods in the box on page 6 does not always cause harm, but it is safer to avoid them.

Your lifestyle

Modify your lifestyle so that you are not excessively tired. If you have a drug habit, this will harm you and your baby. Your doctor can help.

Stop smoking and reduce your alcohol intake so that you are free of these unhealthy habits by the time you fall pregnant. It is amazing how you can do without them and begin to feel better. Do some exercise in moderation. Walking and swimming are gentle and good for your body.

Your health check

Many GPs will arrange for you to have a well woman check before you become pregnant. Your GP may do the check him- or herself, or get the practice nurse to help; some health authorities have their own clinics. In the check you can have a cervical smear and give a blood sample to make sure that you are immune to rubella (German measles) because a woman who catches rubella during early pregnancy may pass the infection on to the developing baby, when it may cause serious defects of the heart, eyes and ears. If your smear is abnormal, you can be treated before you fall pregnant. If your rubella immunity is low, you can be immunised. This will help protect your developing baby.

Age

Most women are between the ages of 20 and 35 when they have babies. If you are older or younger than this, you have a slightly increased risk of complications. Teenagers have smaller babies and give birth prematurely more often, whereas older women have an increased risk of having a baby with an extra chromosome. This is called trisomy, and the most common form is Down syndrome (trisomy 21) (see page 12).

The age-related risk of having a baby with Down syndrome is shown in the box below. The risk begins to increase significantly after the age of 40. A risk of 1 in 200 means that in 199 of 200 instances the outcome is normal.

The only way for a pregnant woman and her doctor to be certain that a baby is not affected by a trisomy is to perform a procedure that provides some of the baby's cells. The two commonly used procedures are chorionic villus sampling (CVS) and amniocentesis, both of which involve making a small puncture in the

Age-related risk of Down syndrome at birth

As women get older, their risk of giving birth to a baby with Down syndrome (trisomy 21) increases. As shown in this table, a woman's risk increases significantly once she passes the age of 40.

Age of mother	Risk of Down syndrome at birth
20 years	1 in 1,500 babies
30 years	1 in 900 babies
35 years	1 in 400 babies
36 years	1 in 250 babies
40 years	1 in 100 babies
45 years	1 in 30 babies
48 years	1 in 10 babies

Adapted from Cuckle et al. (1987) *British Journal of Obstetrics and Gynaecology*, vol. 94, page 387.

Chromosome changes in Down syndrome

Babies with Down syndrome have an extra chromosome 21 in their body's cells (that is, three instead of the normal two).

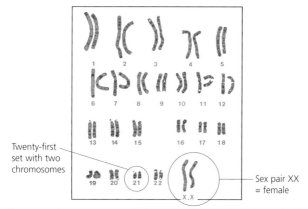

Twenty-first set with two chromosomes

Sex pair XX = female

The normal arrangement of chromosomes in a female. Each of us has 46 chromosomes in the cells of our bodies, made up of 23 pairs. A male would have XY rather than XX in the sex pair (bottom right).

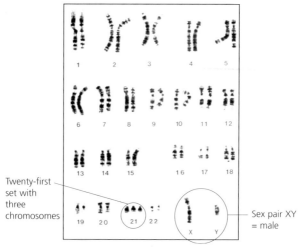

Twenty-first set with three chromosomes

Sex pair XY = male

The arrangement of chromosomes in a male with Down syndrome (trisomy 21). The twenty-first set has three rather than the normal two chromosomes.

membranes around the baby and carry a small risk of causing a miscarriage They are therefore called invasive procedures by contrast with tests that cannot harm the baby such as ultrasound. These procedures are described in detail in 'Screening for fetal abnormality' on page 56.

A trisomy is formed when a problem occurs in the maturation of an egg (oocyte) in the ovary. Each of us has 46 chromosomes in the cells of our body. They are made up of 23 pairs (see figure on page 10) and when the cell divides the chromosomes become visible and can be numbered 1 to 23. One of each pair comes from the sperm of the father and the other from the oocyte or egg of the mother.

Occasionally, an oocyte has 24 chromosomes instead of 23. This does not happen with sperm. An oocyte with an extra chromosome will produce a baby with

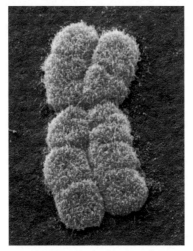

Electron micrograph of a human chromosome.
Chromosomes occur in the nucleus (control centre) of every human cell, carrying genetic information in the form of DNA arranged in segments called genes.

47 chromosomes instead of 46. If the extra chromosome is number 21 then the condition is called trisomy 21 (three copies, not two, of chromosome 21), also known as Down syndrome.

Other trisomies, rarely seen in babies, are trisomy 13 (Patau syndrome) and trisomy 18 (Edward syndrome). Babies with trisomies 13 and 18 have poor growth and many defects affecting the nervous system, the lip and palate, and the internal organs. They do not usually survive for very long after birth and many are stillborn. Most other trisomies affect growth so severely that they result in miscarriage early in pregnancy.

Family history – genetic problems

Some people have a relative who suffers from a physical or mental disorder. Most of these disorders are one-off events that carry no increased risk of happening again. However, you may have a relative who has a genetic problem that runs in the family. If this is the case, you may think that the baby you are carrying may have an increased risk of having a genetic disorder.

It is best to check whether or not you are at risk, especially because some conditions can be tested for in early pregnancy to find out whether or not your developing fetus is affected. Genetic disorders are complex and, if you are at risk, you may need to be referred to a geneticist who can help you understand the condition and predict your risk.

One of the most common parental concerns is when a relative is affected by Down syndrome. Most people who suffer from this condition have trisomy 21. However, one per cent of people with Down syndrome have a different chromosomal abnormality called an 'unbalanced' translocation. During the essential process of reducing by half the number of chromosomes in the sperm and ova, some extra genetic material may be received from the affected parent. This results in the offspring having three chromosome 21s – the two 21 chromosomes that are normally found and the 21 that is attached to 14. If you have a relative who has Down syndrome and you are uncertain whether it is the result of trisomy or an unbalanced translocation, you can have the chromosomes of your white blood cells checked by laboratory examination. If these are normal with no evidence of a translocation, you are at no increased risk.

Single gene disorders

Most genetic problems are carried by a defect in a single gene and so are called single gene disorders. There are thousands of genes on each chromosome. Genetic disorders are classified according to how they are passed on:

- autosomal dominant
- autosomal recessive
- sex (X) linked (see box on pages 14–15 for an explanation of the terms).

The risk to the child varies according to the type of disorder. Many of these can now be diagnosed in early pregnancy.

Genetic and environmental causes

Some abnormalities that occur may be the result of a combination of genetic and environmental factors and are termed 'multi-factorial' in origin. Spina bifida is a

Single gene disorders

Single gene disorders (when only one gene has a defect) can be passed on in three different ways.

Autosomal dominant
All the individuals who have the abnormal gene are affected, but because genes come in pairs they will pass the abnormal gene on to only half of their children, and each child will have a one in two chance of inheriting the abnormal gene and the disease, and a one in two chance of being unaffected.

Examples of autosomal dominant gene disorders

- Huntington's disease (causes abnormal movements and mental deterioration in later life)
- Myotonic dystrophy (causes muscle weakness)

Autosomal recessive
Individuals with one abnormal gene are unaffected, but if both parents have the same abnormal gene each of their children will have a one in four risk of inheriting a double dose of the abnormal gene and so of having the disease.

Examples of autosomal recessive gene disorders

- Cystic fibrosis (problems with lungs and digestive system)
- Sickle-cell disease (blood disorder causing anaemia and painful 'crises')
- Thalassaemia (blood disorder causing anaemia and slow growth)

physical defect present at birth which results in weakness or paralysis of the legs and poor bladder and bowel control resulting from a poorly formed spine and spinal cord. It is an example of such a condition

Single gene disorders (contd)

X-linked

The abnormal gene is on an X chromosome.
Females have two X chromosomes (one affected,
one not) and do not usually develop the disease.
They always pass an X chromosome to a male child
and so there is a 50 per cent chance that he will
inherit the affected X. If a male inherits the abnormal
gene he will develop the disease. All his female
children will be carriers of the abnormal gene and
none of his sons will be affected.

Examples of X-linked gene disorders

- Duchenne muscular dystrophy (causes progressive
  muscle weakness)
- Haemophilia (blood disorder in which blood is
  slow to clot)

where genetics and vitamin (folic acid) deficiency have
a combined role in causing the disorder.

Twenty-five years ago, this condition occurred in one
in 200 pregnancies but, with improving diet and folic
acid supplementation, the risk is now one in 500. If a
woman has a pregnancy affected by spina bifida, the
risk of recurrence in a subsequent pregnancy is
increased to one in 20. With high-dose folic acid (5 mg
daily) before conception and for the first 12 weeks of
pregnancy, this risk is reduced by almost 80 per cent.

Medical history

Pre-pregnancy counselling is advisable if you suffer
from diabetes or epilepsy. Strict control of blood sugar
in the first few weeks of pregnancy in women with
diabetes has been clearly shown to reduce the risk of

miscarriage and fetal abnormality. So your insulin type and dosage require close medical supervision.

If you suffer from epilepsy, you should not stop your medication without discussing this with your doctor. Some of the anti-epileptic drugs are safer for the developing fetus and it may be possible to change to one of these under medical supervision. Recurrent seizures may deprive your developing baby of oxygen and cause harm. Some of the anti-epileptic drugs are associated with a slight increase in the risk of spina bifida and heart defects. It is important to take folic acid 5 mg daily to reduce the risk. If you haven't had a seizure for two years, you may no longer require medication but your doctor should advise you on how to reduce and stop your drugs.

Medical disorders and pregnancy

Some medical disorders can cause problems during pregnancy, affecting the development of the baby, the health of the mother or both:

- Blood clotting disorders
- Deep vein thrombosis
- Diabetes
- Epilepsy
- Heart problem
- High blood pressure
- Persistent infection
- Previous pulmonary embolism
- Psychiatric disorder
- Thyroid disorders

Some other medical disorders (see box) may complicate a pregnancy. Some disorders improve with pregnancy, some get worse and others remain unchanged.

Involve your doctor

If you are on medication, it is important for your doctor to know that you are planning a pregnancy because some drugs such as isotretinoin taken for acne must not be taken during the early months of pregnancy. The most critical time for the development of the organs of the developing baby (known as an 'embryo' at this time) is between three and five weeks after conception. This is five to seven weeks after the first day of your last menstrual period and is known as the period of organogenesis or embryogenesis. It is better to avoid unnecessary medication during this time.

KEY POINTS

- If you have a medical condition or a family history of a genetic disorder, you may need specialised pre-pregnancy counselling

- Take folic acid (400 micrograms daily) before conception and for 12 weeks after your last period

- Modify your lifestyle to stop smoking, reduce alcohol intake and improve your diet

- If you have a drug habit, you are likely to be addicted. See your doctor for advice

- Unless you have a significant illness, investigate avoiding medication during the period of organogenesis (when the baby's organs develop – from five to seven weeks after the first day of your last period)

Fertilisation and development of the fetus and placenta

The menstrual cycle

The average length of the menstrual cycle is 28 days and the first day of the menstrual period is referred to as day 1 of the cycle. Release of an egg from the ovary (ovulation) normally takes place around day 14 and the interval between ovulation and the onset of menstruation is usually fixed at 14 days. During the menstrual cycle there are various hormones at work and these are necessary to cause the ovary to release an egg (oocyte) and to prepare the lining of the uterus (endometrium) for a developing embryo. Several hormones are involved in this process, as follows.

Follicle-stimulating hormone

Follicle-stimulating hormone (FSH) is produced from the pituitary gland, which lies at the base of the brain. Each month it stimulates the growth and ripening of between 5 and 12 oocytes within their follicles

The menstrual cycle

Each month from puberty to the menopause a woman's body goes through the menstrual cycle. The cycle is controlled by the interaction of four hormones, affecting the ovaries and the release of mature eggs and the wall of the uterus (endometrium).

Menstruation **Preovulation** **Ovulation** **Postovulation**

The principal changes in hormones over the menstrual cycle

FSH causes an egg follicle to start developing in the ovary

Oestrogen stimulates the lining of the uterus to thicken. The level peaks just before ovulation

Around mid-cycle a surge of LH triggers ovulation

Progesterone continues the thickening of the uterine wall for the fertilised egg to implant into

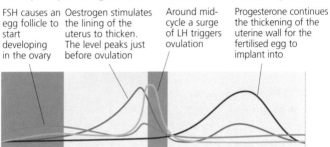

Eggs develop in the ovaries before being released into the fallopian tubes and travelling to the uterus

Egg starts to grow in the follicle, stimulated by FSH

Developing egg

Follicle ruptures, mature egg released into fallopian tube

Corpus luteum formed from empty follicle

Corpus luteum shrinks and dies

The changes in the lining of the uterus over the menstrual cycle

Menstrual bleeding

Unfertilised egg from last menstrual cycle leaves uterus

Endometrium (lining of the uterus) doubles in thickness, in response to hormones

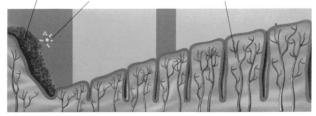

(fluid-filled swellings in the ovaries). Peak secretion of FSH coincides with an oocyte reaching maturity. FSH also aids the release of the oocyte into the fallopian tube. The amount secreted then falls back to the baseline level. Each ovary has around 20,000 oocytes at puberty but fewer than 12 are stimulated at the beginning of each menstrual cycle. Of these only one usually develops into a mature follicle which releases an oocyte at ovulation in the middle of the menstrual cycle.

Luteinising hormone

Luteinising hormone (LH), like FSH, is produced by the pituitary gland. There is a surge in LH blood levels just before ovulation and this results in the final maturation and release of the oocyte from the follicle. LH then acts on the cells within the follicle to convert it to the corpus luteum, the cavity left when the follicle has ruptured. The corpus luteum secretes the hormones oestrogen and progesterone, preparing the lining of the uterus to receive the newly fertilised ovum.

Oestrogen

This hormone is produced by the cells in the follicle and corpus luteum and brings about the changes that occur in the endometrium. Its level rises and falls in the first half of the cycle and reaches a second, smaller peak again in the second half. During the first half, it causes the endometrium to thicken and, in the second half, along with progesterone, it maintains the endometrium in its spongy, secretory phase in which glands in the endometrium enlarge and start to secrete nutrients for the possible embryo.

Progesterone

This hormone is produced in the second half of the menstrual cycle by the corpus luteum and brings about the development of the secretory endometrium, so that it is ready to receive and nourish a fertilised oocyte. The blood level of this hormone can be measured on day 21 of the cycle to confirm that ovulation has occurred.

If fertilisation fails to occur, the corpus luteum degenerates. Consequently, oestrogen and progesterone production decreases and the endometrium is no longer supported. Menstruation then occurs with the shedding of the endometrium.

Conception and the first journey of life

An oocyte is normally fertilised by a single, one-celled sperm 12 to 24 hours after it is released. Oocytes and sperm each have 23 chromosomes, and when a sperm penetrates an oocyte its chromosomes can move freely. The chromosomes from the sperm and the oocyte then pair up to make cells of 46 chromosomes. Conception has occurred.

After about 36 hours the fertilised oocyte divides into two cells and by three days it has multiplied to 12 to 16 cells and is known as a morula (mulberry). The morula is wafted down through the fallopian tube and on day 7 enters the cavity of the uterus. Its development continues and some fluid appears inside it, making it look like a cyst. It is now called a blastocyst and it implants into the endometrium (the lining of the wall of the uterus) on day 9 (see figure on page 24).

Fertilisation

Of about 100 million sperm that are ejaculated, only around 500 to 1,000 remain by the time they reach the egg at the outer end of the fallopian tube. Only one sperm penetrates the egg to cause fertilisation.

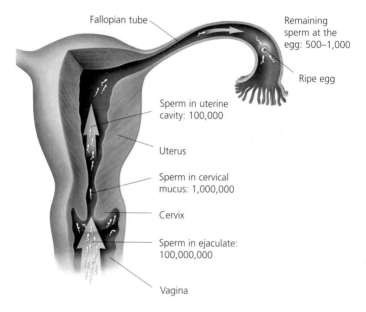

Fallopian tube

Remaining sperm at the egg: 500–1,000

Ripe egg

Sperm in uterine cavity: 100,000

Uterus

Sperm in cervical mucus: 1,000,000

Cervix

Sperm in ejaculate: 100,000,000

Vagina

Embryo formation

Under the influence of progesterone and oestrogen secreted from the corpus luteum, the glands and blood vessels in the endometrium have developed so that it has become spongy and ready to receive the blastocyst, which by then is termed the 'embryo'.

By day 14, the embryo is completely embedded and the implantation site in the endometrium heals over. When the implantation site is sealed, there is sometimes a little bleeding and this show of blood may be mistaken for a period. This sometimes explains why some pregnancies are later found to be a month further on than thought.

Implantation

The fertilised egg divides rapidly, first to form a morula and then a blastocyst. After about six to seven days, the blastocyst reaches the uterine cavity where it implants in the endometrium.

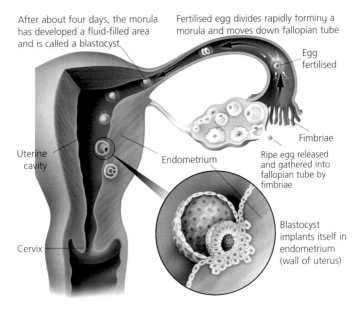

After about four days, the morula has developed a fluid-filled area and is called a blastocyst

Fertilised egg divides rapidly forming a morula and moves down fallopian tube

Egg fertilised

Fimbriae

Uterine cavity

Endometrium

Ripe egg released and gathered into fallopian tube by fimbriae

Cervix

Blastocyst implants itself in endometrium (wall of uterus)

Ectopic pregnancy

Occasionally this early journey for the morula may be delayed. Sometimes there is no obvious reason for the delay but it may be caused by a blockage or adhesions in the tiny bore of the fallopian tube. This can be a result of a past infection which may or may not have been obvious to the patient.

When this delay occurs, the morula fails to reach the uterine cavity. However, it continues to develop and implants in an abnormal (ectopic) site usually within the wall of the fallopian tube. This becomes an ectopic pregnancy (see figure opposite) and it cannot survive

Types of ectopic pregnancy

An ectopic pregnancy occurs where the fertilised ovum implants outside of the uterine cavity, and is usually unable to continue to term.

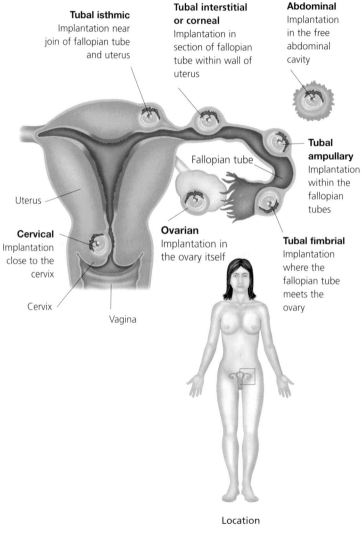

Tubal isthmic
Implantation near join of fallopian tube and uterus

Tubal interstitial or corneal
Implantation in section of fallopian tube within wall of uterus

Abdominal
Implantation in the free abdominal cavity

Fallopian tube

Tubal ampullary
Implantation within the fallopian tubes

Uterus

Cervical
Implantation close to the cervix

Ovarian
Implantation in the ovary itself

Tubal fimbrial
Implantation where the fallopian tube meets the ovary

Cervix

Vagina

Location

because the site of implantation is too weak to support the developing pregnancy.

Rupture of the ectopic pregnancy may occur, sometimes with severe internal bleeding (see 'Pregnancy loss', page 160). Very rarely the pregnancy may implant among the pelvic organs and continue as an abdominal pregnancy, but this hardly ever reaches a size and maturity to allow surgical delivery.

Placenta formation

When the blastocyst attaches to the endometrium (wall of the uterus) on day 9, it has an inner mass of cells which develops into the embryo and an outer mass of cells that are called trophoblasts (see figure opposite). The trophoblast cells begin to develop their own blood supply and this outer cell mass becomes known as the chorion which later develops into the placenta (or afterbirth).

The cells produce a hormone called human chorionic gonadotrophin (hCG) and this is the hormone that is detected in a pregnancy test. It is first produced in very small amounts and can be detected by sensitive tests at the time of your first missed period.

The embryo and formation of the organs

By day 14 after the release of the oocyte, the trophoblast is completely embedded and the inner cells begin to line up as two layers of different cells (see figure on page 28). Pregnancy is now suspected because of the missed period. Doctors and midwives refer to the number of weeks after the first day of your last period as the gestational age of your pregnancy (and this dating of the pregnancy will be used from this point in the book).

Human blastocyst at nine days

The blastocyst starts to embed itself into the wall of the uterus (implantation). Its inner cells begin to develop into an embryo, while the outer cells begin to form the placenta.

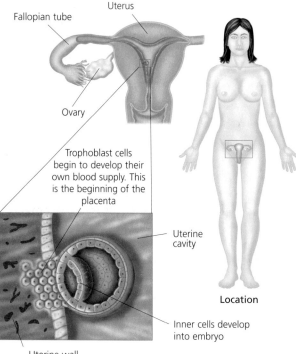

Fallopian tube

Uterus

Ovary

Trophoblast cells begin to develop their own blood supply. This is the beginning of the placenta

Uterine cavity

Location

Inner cells develop into embryo

Uterine wall

The cell differentiation continues and, as early as five weeks (from the last period), the inner mass of cells begins to change into tissues and organs. Tissues include skin and bones and the basic cells responsible for these are laid down. Organs include the brain, heart, eyes and ears, and these are formed by the end of nine weeks after the last menstrual period.

Using pregnancy ultrasound scanning, the blastocyst is seen as a small circle measuring two to four millimetres

Human embryo at two weeks

By day 14, the embryo is completely embedded into the uterus. It measures about 0.2 millimetre and has no nervous system or organs.

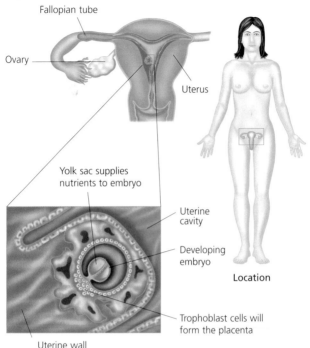

Fallopian tube

Ovary

Uterus

Yolk sac supplies nutrients to embryo

Uterine cavity

Developing embryo

Location

Trophoblast cells will form the placenta

Uterine wall

within the uterus at 4.5 weeks after your last period. The first pulsations of the heart beat can be seen as early as 36 days after the last period when the embryo measures only two to four millimetres. The yolk sac is seen close to the embryo and measures about 10 mm.

The gestation period from week 5 to the end of week 9 is called the embryonic period or period of organogenesis. This is a vital time for development of the organs – most abnormalities or defects that are found after birth have happened during this time. We know this from case studies

Human embryo at three weeks

The embryo is now well established inside the amniotic sac (for protection) with a food supply (yolk sac). The placenta is formed and working. The embryo measures about three millimetres in length.

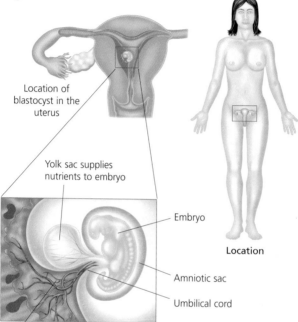

Location of blastocyst in the uterus

Yolk sac supplies nutrients to embryo

Embryo

Amniotic sac

Umbilical cord

Placenta

Location

of patients who have had rubella (German measles). The most damaging effects occur when a mother has the illness between week 5 and week 7 of the gestation period – her baby may be born blind, deaf and with heart defects.

Rubella is caused by a virus and because it can cause birth defects it is called a teratogen. Certain drugs have teratogenic properties (the best known are thalidomide and the retinoids) and should be avoided during the period of organogenesis. Most medications should be avoided at this time except supplements such as folic acid

Human embryo at four weeks

The embryo measures about four to five millimetres in length. Its internal organs, head, eyes and limbs are beginning to form.

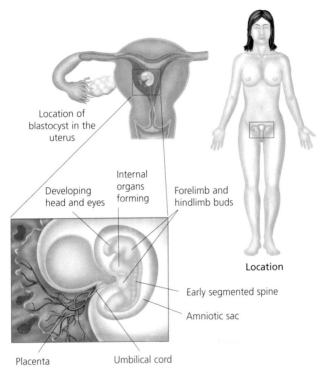

Location of blastocyst in the uterus

Developing head and eyes

Internal organs forming

Forelimb and hindlimb buds

Location

Early segmented spine

Amniotic sac

Placenta

Umbilical cord

or others that may be vital for your health. Although most birth defects occur during the period of organogenesis, the cause is not usually known. The formation of the embryo is a series of complex biological events and occasionally things go wrong. Some abnormalities may be lethal – the embryo dies and miscarriage results.

The fetus

By the beginning of 10 weeks' gestation, the outline of a baby becomes recognisable and it is now called a fetus. Organ formation is almost complete and the fetus now starts to mature and prepare for delivery at around 40 weeks from the last period. The skin initially appears red and transparent but progressively thickens in the last few weeks when it is covered in a layer of white grease called vernix. This prevents the mature skin becoming crinkly and waterlogged while bathed in amniotic fluid in the uterus.

The sex is recognisable on external appearance by 14 weeks, although the actual sex was determined at conception. If you have an ultrasound scan at this time it is rather early to be certain of the sex but usually at the time of the 20-week scan it is possible, depending on how your fetus is lying.

At 10 weeks the fetus weighs only 10 grams and measures 3 centimetres (cm) from the top of the head to the base of the spine (crown–rump length). Growth is considerable over the next 30 weeks and the average weight at delivery is 3,500 grams (7.5 pounds) when the crown–rump length is 35 cm (see box on page 32). The body proportions also change over this period. At 10 weeks, the head size is about half the crown–rump length, but by 40 weeks it is only about a quarter because of the increase in size of the trunk.

The fetus becomes viable at 24 weeks. This means that it is possible for it to survive if delivered after this time. However, delivery at 24 weeks is very hazardous for a newborn because the organs and tissues are still very immature. The chance of survival is not good and, if survival does occur, the chance of handicap is high. As each week passes beyond the 24-week gestational age of viability, the chances of intact survival increase greatly. With modern neonatal care, most babies will survive after 30 weeks.

Fetal weight and length changes

The developing baby's weight and length increase
throughout the pregnancy:

Weeks of pregnancy	Fetal weight (grams)	Crown–rump length (cm)
10 weeks	10 g	3 cm
22 weeks	500 g	20 cm
28 weeks	1,000 g	25 cm
40 weeks	3,500 g	35 cm

Changes in the baby's proportions

As the pregnancy progresses, the developing baby grows rapidly.
This shows the relative changes in fetal size and proportions
between week 8 and week 22 of pregnancy.

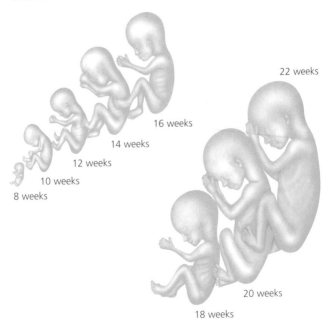

22 weeks

16 weeks

14 weeks

12 weeks

10 weeks

8 weeks

20 weeks

18 weeks

The placenta

When the trophoblast invades the endometrium it develops tiny stems and branches. Within these, blood vessels form and develop into a network resulting in the formation of the chorion. At around 10 weeks the chorionic development is concentrated in the area nearest the fetus (see figure below). It becomes the true placenta and its circulation links up with the fetus through the connecting stalk, which becomes the umbilical cord. The chorion has the same genetic make-up as the fetus and it can be sampled at this stage in pregnancy for the prenatal diagnosis of specific genetic or chromosome problems.

The chorion (precursor of the placenta)

At around 10 weeks, the chorionic villi grow into the uterine wall, near the fetus, and establish an intimate connection with the mother's own blood vessels. This becomes the true placenta and links to the fetus via the umbilical cord. The placenta can develop anywhere on the uterine wall, not only in the position seen in this diagram.

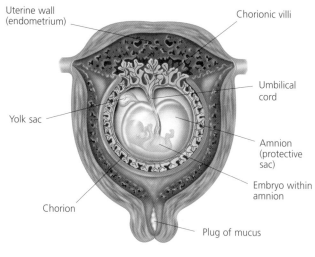

Uterine wall (endometrium)

Chorionic villi

Umbilical cord

Yolk sac

Amnion (protective sac)

Embryo within amnion

Chorion

Plug of mucus

The placenta

The fetus is reliant on the mother for oxygen and nutrients.
The placenta allows the exchange of oxygen and nourishment
from the mother to the fetus.

Cross-section through placenta

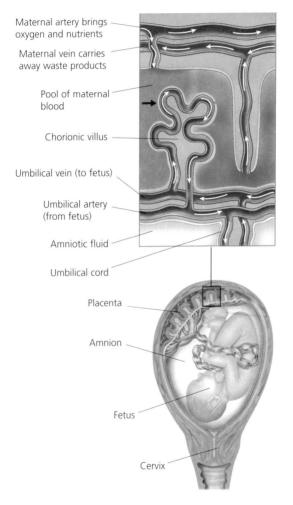

Maternal artery brings oxygen and nutrients

Maternal vein carries away waste products

Pool of maternal blood

Chorionic villus

Umbilical vein (to fetus)

Umbilical artery (from fetus)

Amniotic fluid

Umbilical cord

Placenta

Amnion

Fetus

Cervix

The tiny stems and their branches are called villi and these chorionic villi erode the tiny blood vessels in the endometrium. They become bathed by the mother's blood and from this oxygen and nutrients pass across the thin barrier of cells from the mother to the blood in the placenta, and then onto the fetus through the umbilical cord. The uteroplacental circulation has become established (see figure) and the developing fetus is dependent on its mother for nutrition. The placenta also produces hormones, which aid the growth of the fetus and maintain the pregnancy.

KEY POINTS

- The average length of the menstrual cycle is 28 days and ovulation occurs 14 days before the onset of menstruation

- FSH and LH from the pituitary gland cause ovulation

- Oestrogen and progesterone from the corpus luteum prepare the secretory endometrium for the fertilised egg

- Detection of human chorionic gonadotrophin in the mother's urine or blood confirms that conception has occurred

- The embryonic period, when the organs form, lasts from five to nine weeks after the first day of the last period

- The fetal period lasts from 10 weeks until delivery at about 40 weeks

Confirmation of pregnancy and routine tests

The pregnancy test

You should know when your period is overdue. To confirm that you are pregnant it is simple to do a pregnancy test. The basis of this test is to detect the hormone, human chorionic gonadotrophin (hCG), in your urine. As mentioned in the previous chapter, this is produced by the chorionic villi very early in pregnancy.

Chorionic villi start to grow only *when the oocyte has been fertilised*. The hCG is produced only by the chorionic villi and no other tissue, so it is specific. It is detectable in your blood and urine. It is present in very small amounts in your circulation at the time of the missed period. The level doubles every two to three days, reaches a peak at ten weeks and then falls.

Pregnancy testing kits (see figure on page 39) can be bought from a pharmacist, or it may be possible for you to be tested at your doctor's surgery or at a family

Range of serum hCG values

The hormone human chorionic gonadotrophin (hCG) can be detected in your urine very early on in the pregnancy. By the first day of the missed period, the hCG levels are rising rapidly.

Days after last menstrual period	Serum hCG range (international units per millilitre of urine or IU/l)
30	200–5,000 IU/l
40	9,000–48,000 IU/l
60	35,000–95,000 IU/l
70	48,000–100,000 IU/l

planning clinic. The result of the test is 99 per cent accurate but it is best to check it on two separate occasions, two to three days apart.

You can test your urine a few days after your missed period. If you do it too soon after your missed period your hCG level may be too low to be detectable in your urine. It is best to use the first urine passed in the morning because this is the most concentrated.

Reliable kits will yield positive results when the urine level is as low as 25 international units per litre (IU/l). In some women this level is found two to three days before the expected period. By the first day of the missed period, concentrations often exceed 100 IU/l.

Your menstrual history

If you are planning a pregnancy, you should mark in a diary the days when you have your period. The first day of your period is important to note because it is

Home pregnancy tests

A home pregnancy testing kit confirms pregnancy if it detects hCG, a hormone in your urine that is produced very early in pregnancy. Pregnancy tests vary in how they portray a positive result. In this example, a positive result is shown by crossed lines in the result indicator window on the testing device.

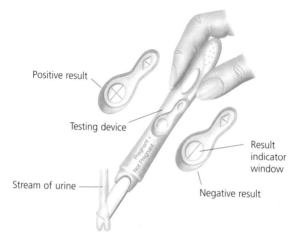

Positive result

Testing device

Stream of urine

Result indicator window

Negative result

regarded as day 1 of your menstrual cycle. You can then work out what your normal cycle is. Most women have a cycle of 28 days, which means that there are 28 days from the beginning of one period to the beginning of the next.

As the interval between ovulation and the first day of a period is usually 14 days, you will ovulate on day 14 if you have a 28-day cycle. Your best chance of falling pregnant is to have sex on the day that you ovulate or two to three days before or after. Ovulation prediction kits can be bought from pharmacies to test for the surge in luteinising hormone (LH) in your urine which marks ovulation (see 'Fertilisation and development of the fetus and placenta', page 19).

Some women have irregular cycles and others have

long or short cycles. Those with irregular cycles are less likely to be ovulating regularly. Those with long or short cycles will usually ovulate 14 days before their expected period. This means that a woman who has a 35-day cycle will normally ovulate on day 21 of her cycle. On the other hand, a woman with a 24-day cycle will ovulate on day 10.

Calculating your due date

When you fall pregnant, you will be asked when the first day of your last menstrual period (LMP) was. It is very helpful for the medical and midwifery staff because they can then calculate your expected date of delivery (EDD). The average length of pregnancy is 40 weeks from the LMP, the normal range being 38 to 42 weeks.

Calculation of expected date of delivery (EDD)

Midwives and other medical staff can calculate your EDD by taking into account the date of your last menstrual perion (LMP).

Assuming that you have a 28-day cycle, the rule is to add 7 days to your LMP and then subtract 3 months.

LMP is 3 February
Add 7 days to 3 February = 10 February
Subtract 3 months from 10 February = 10 November
Therefore EDD is 10 November

LMP is 30 July
Add 7 days to 30 July = 6 August (there are 31 days in July)
Subtract 3 months from 6 August = 6 May
Therefore EDD is 6 May

So your EDD will be 40 weeks from your LMP. There are pregnancy calculators that can work out your due date but there is a simple method that you can do in your head or with the help of a calendar. From the date of the month, add seven days and, from the actual month, subtract three months. There are some examples in the box. The chart on pages 42–3 can help you determine your EDD without any calculations.

The calculation and chart assume that you have a 28-day cycle. If you have a 35-day cycle you have to add another 7 days to your EDD because ovulation occurs 7 days later than in a 28-day cycle. If your last period occurred when you stopped the pill, your normal cycle and ovulation may not have been established so the calculations may not be accurate. Sometimes you may have vaginal bleeding when you are already pregnant and this can mimic a period and again give you the wrong estimate. For these reasons doctors tend to rely on ultrasound scanning to assess the gestational age of your pregnancy.

Your booking visit

When you have missed a period and your pregnancy test is positive, you will need to telephone your doctor's surgery to make an appointment for pregnancy care. You will probably know where you want your baby to be born and whether he or she will be delivered by a hospital doctor, a midwife or your GP.

Arrangements will be made for you to see your doctor, practice nurse or midwife and you may be referred to the local maternity hospital for booking. This simply means that you are being booked at a specific maternity (obstetrics) unit, which in many cases you can choose or at least have a preference, and that your pregnancy care will be supervised according to their guidelines.

Calculating your date for delivery

To calculate your expected date of delivery, find the date of the first day of your last menstrual period on the top (blue)

January	1	2	3	4	5	6	7	8	9	10	11	12	13	14	15	16
October	8	9	10	11	12	13	14	15	16	17	18	19	20	21	22	23

February	1	2	3	4	5	6	7	8	9	10	11	12	13	14	15	16
November	8	9	10	11	12	13	14	15	16	17	18	19	20	21	22	23

March	1	2	3	4	5	6	7	8	9	10	11	12	13	14	15	16
December	6	7	8	9	10	11	12	13	14	15	16	17	18	19	20	21

April	1	2	3	4	5	6	7	8	9	10	11	12	13	14	15	16
January	6	7	8	9	10	11	12	13	14	15	16	17	18	19	20	21

May	1	2	3	4	5	6	7	8	9	10	11	12	13	14	15	16
February	5	6	7	8	9	10	11	12	13	14	15	16	17	18	19	20

June	1	2	3	4	5	6	7	8	9	10	11	12	13	14	15	16
March	8	9	10	11	12	13	14	15	16	17	18	19	20	21	22	23

July	1	2	3	4	5	6	7	8	9	10	11	12	13	14	15	16
April	7	8	9	10	11	12	13	14	15	16	17	18	19	20	21	22

August	1	2	3	4	5	6	7	8	9	10	11	12	13	14	15	16
May	8	9	10	11	12	13	14	15	16	17	18	19	20	21	22	23

September	1	2	3	4	5	6	7	8	9	10	11	12	13	14	15	16
June	8	9	10	11	12	13	14	15	16	17	18	19	20	21	22	23

October	1	2	3	4	5	6	7	8	9	10	11	12	13	14	15	16
July	8	9	10	11	12	13	14	15	16	17	18	19	20	21	22	23

November	1	2	3	4	5	6	7	8	9	10	11	12	13	14	15	16
August	8	9	10	11	12	13	14	15	16	17	18	19	20	21	22	23

December	1	2	3	4	5	6	7	8	9	10	11	12	13	14	15	16
September	7	8	9	10	11	12	13	14	15	16	17	18	19	20	21	22

line of the chart. The date immediately below this is your expected date of delivery.

17	**18**	**19**	**20**	**21**	**22**	**23**	**24**	**25**	**26**	**27**	**28**	**29**	**30**	**31**	**January**
24	25	26	27	28	29	30	31	1	2	3	4	5	6	7	November

17	**18**	**19**	**20**	**21**	**22**	**23**	**24**	**25**	**26**	**27**	**28**				**February**
24	25	26	27	28	29	30	1	2	3	4	5				December

17	**18**	**19**	**20**	**21**	**22**	**23**	**24**	**25**	**26**	**27**	**28**	**29**	**30**	**31**	**March**
22	23	24	25	26	27	28	29	30	31	1	2	3	4	5	January

17	**18**	**19**	**20**	**21**	**22**	**23**	**24**	**25**	**26**	**27**	**28**	**29**	**30**		**April**
22	23	24	25	26	27	28	29	30	31	1	2	3	4		February

17	**18**	**19**	**20**	**21**	**22**	**23**	**24**	**25**	**26**	**27**	**28**	**29**	**30**	**31**	**May**
21	22	23	24	25	26	27	28	1	2	3	4	5	6	7	March

17	**18**	**19**	**20**	**21**	**22**	**23**	**24**	**25**	**26**	**27**	**28**	**29**	**30**		**June**
24	25	26	27	28	29	30	31	1	2	3	4	5	6		April

17	**18**	**19**	**20**	**21**	**22**	**23**	**24**	**25**	**26**	**27**	**28**	**29**	**30**	**31**	**July**
23	24	25	26	27	28	29	30	1	2	3	4	5	6	7	May

17	**18**	**19**	**20**	**21**	**22**	**23**	**24**	**25**	**26**	**27**	**28**	**29**	**30**	**31**	**August**
24	25	26	27	28	29	30	31	1	2	3	4	5	6	7	June

17	**18**	**19**	**20**	**21**	**22**	**23**	**24**	**25**	**26**	**27**	**28**	**29**	**30**		**September**
24	25	26	27	28	29	30	1	2	3	4	5	6	7		July

17	**18**	**19**	**20**	**21**	**22**	**23**	**24**	**25**	**26**	**27**	**28**	**29**	**30**	**31**	**October**
24	25	26	27	28	29	30	31	1	2	3	4	5	6	7	August

17	**18**	**19**	**20**	**21**	**22**	**23**	**24**	**25**	**26**	**27**	**28**	**29**	**30**		**November**
24	25	26	27	28	29	30	31	1	2	3	4	5	6		September

17	**18**	**19**	**20**	**21**	**22**	**23**	**24**	**25**	**26**	**27**	**28**	**29**	**30**	**31**	**December**
23	24	25	26	27	28	29	30	1	2	3	4	5	6	7	October

Cases requiring hospital referral

There are several reasons why a mother may need to be referred to a consultant clinic at a hospital. She may have a specific medical condition or family history, a problem with one of her previous pregnancies or a problem relating to her current pregnancy.

Medical condition
- Diabetes/endocrine disorder
- Epilepsy
- Renal disease
- Genetic problem
- Previous psychiatric illness
- High blood pressure (hypertension)
- Blood disorder
- Heart disease
- Previous uterine surgery
- Other serious disorder

Previous obstetric problem
- Recurrent miscarriage
- Low birthweight (less than 2.5 kg)
- Caesarean section
- Fetal abnormality
- Significant bleeding after delivery (postpartum haemorrhage)
- Pre-term labour (before 37 weeks)
- Severe pregnancy-induced high blood pressure (pre-eclampsia, see page 100)
- Difficult delivery

Cases requiring hospital referral (contd)

- Stillbirth or birth-related illness or death in first year
- Damage in earlier pregnancy to perineum (area between vagina and anus)

Factors relating to this pregnancy

- Younger than 16
- Low haemoglobin – less than 100 grams/litre (< 100 g/l)
- Hepatitis carrier
- Substance misuse
- More than one embryo/fetus
- Older than 37, first pregnancy
- Blood group antibodies present in blood
- HIV positive
- Amniocentesis/CVS (screening results indicating elevated risk)
- Some concern that leads to a request to be seen by consultant

A maternity case record is started which will record your relevant medical history and any particular features that may complicate your pregnancy. In most individuals there are no risk factors and antenatal care can be undertaken by midwives and/or general practitioners. In some women there are risk factors that may complicate the pregnancy. If you have any of these you will be referred to the consultant clinic at the maternity hospital.

At your booking visit to the hospital, an early ultrasound scan may be done and various blood tests taken.

The early pregnancy ultrasound scan

Obstetric ultrasound was developed after experience with metal flaw detectors. It obtains images of the uterus and fetus by sending sound waves through the skin and presenting the reflections on a screen or a series of photographic prints.

In the past 30 years millions of babies have had scans and the results monitored. This has shown that ultrasound has no unwanted side effects and does no harm to the fetus.

An ultrasound scan in the first three months of pregnancy (the first trimester) is a very useful clinical investigation. It is done by a sonographer. It has three main purposes – to establish the viability, the gestational age and the number of fetuses.

Viability of a pregnancy

A pregnancy is considered viable once the fetal heart beat has been seen. The earliest gestation at which this can be seen is 5.5 weeks and a transvaginal scan probe may be required for this. If the fluid-filled egg-shaped sac containing the embryo measures more than 20 millimetres in diameter and there is no evidence of cell multiplication at the site that the embryo should develop or heart pulsation, it is highly likely that the pregnancy has developed without an obvious embryo. This is called an anembryonic pregnancy and usually the embryo has died at a very early stage before it is visible on scan. This is discussed further under 'Pregnancy loss' (page 160).

Gestation age

The gestational age can be assessed, with accuracy, to within a week in the first trimester, by measurement of

Ultrasound scans

In the first three months of pregnancy, an ultrasound scan is used to check the viability of the pregnancy, the gestational age (to determine the estimated date of delivery or EDD) and the number of developing babies.

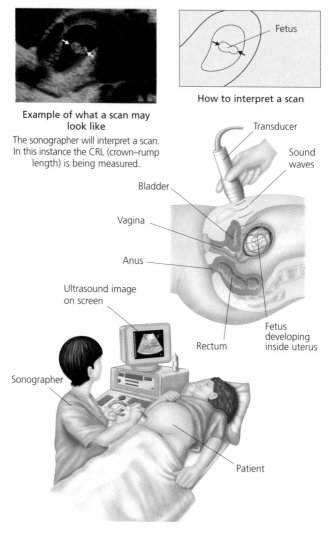

Example of what a scan may look like

The sonographer will interpret a scan. In this instance the CRL (crown–rump length) is being measured.

Fetus

How to interpret a scan

Transducer

Sound waves

Bladder

Vagina

Anus

Ultrasound image on screen

Fetus developing inside uterus

Rectum

Sonographer

Patient

the crown–rump length (CRL). At this time, there is very little biological variation in the CRL measurement between fetuses. This means that, for a given measurement, the gestational age can be calculated to within three days. The CRL increases quite dramatically from week to week and so differences are easily seen and measured (see figure on page 47). In this way, an accurate estimate of the gestational age can be obtained. It may be that your due date (estimated date of delivery or EDD) calculated from your LMP will be changed, based on the CRL measurement. If there is no heart pulsation in a fetus where the CRL is more than six millimetres, the pregnancy is not viable. This means that, sadly, the fetus has died (for reasons frequently unknown). This is discussed further under 'Pregnancy loss' (page 160).

Number of fetuses

The sonographer will scan your whole uterus from top to bottom and from left to right, to make sure that you have only one fetus. In 1 in 80 pregnancies there are 2 and, in 1 in 1,600, there are 3! If you have twins it is useful at this time to identify whether each fetus has a separate placenta (dichorionic) or a shared placenta (monochorionic). Monochorionic twins are always identical but only around 30 per cent of dichorionic twins will be identical. When the placenta is shared there is a greater risk that one fetus will obtain more nutrition than the other and you will need more frequent follow-up scans.

Many hospitals now try to see patients for booking at 11 to 14 weeks, as at this time the nuchal translucency (the skinfold thickness behind the neck of the fetus) can also be measured (see 'Screening for fetal abnormality', page 56).

Blood tests and other investigations

Several investigations are undertaken routinely on your first visit to the GP, obstetrician or midwife who will be monitoring your progress, and some may be repeated later in pregnancy (see box on page 50). Other investigations may be performed if required. You should be aware of these so that you know what it means for you if a result is abnormal.

Haemoglobin

Your blood count is measured to check your haemoglobin (Hb) level to make sure that you are not anaemic. The level will be low (< 100 g/l) if your diet lacks sufficient iron and/or folic acid (see 'Planning a pregnancy', page 1). In some areas of the UK and in many countries of the world, an iron supplement is given routinely to prevent the development of iron deficiency anaemia. Sometimes, during pregnancy, your Hb level falls because there is not enough iron and folic acid in your body for the development of the fetus and placenta. You will need to take iron and/or folic acid if your Hb level is too low.

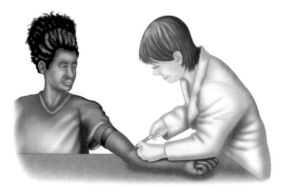

Some blood samples will be taken to assess your general health and other specific factors.

Laboratory tests

Several laboratory investigations are performed to monitor the progress of the mother and check that she remains in good health. Some of these tests may be repeated during the pregnancy at specific intervals.

Test	Test type	Timing
Full blood count	Blood test	Booking, 28 weeks, 36 weeks
Haemoglobin electrophoresis for genetic disorders	Blood test	Booking
Blood group	Blood test	Booking, 28 weeks
Blood group antibodies	Blood test	Booking and as advised by laboratory
Rubella	Blood test	Booking (and after contact with infection if not immune)
Hepatitis B and C	Blood test	Booking
HIV status	Blood test	Booking (you can refuse – see page 53)
Syphilis testing	Blood test	Booking
Glucose and protein in urine	Urine sample	Every visit
Blood glucose	Blood test	28 weeks
Urine specimen for culture	Urine sample	As required
Blood screening for Down syndrome	Blood test	12 and/or 16 weeks
Blood screening for spina bifida	Blood test	16 weeks
Cervical smear	Smear test	As required

Inherited blood disorders

Other tests on your blood such as haemoglobin electrophoresis may be required if you have a family history of the inherited blood disorder thalassaemia or sickle-cell disease. Thalassaemias are more common in those people of Mediterranean, Asian or Oriental extraction. Sickle-cell disease is more common in those of African–Caribbean or Asian origin. These disorders are caused by genetic variations in the red pigment haemoglobin. If you are a carrier of one of these conditions, your partner will need to be tested, but if his haemoglobin is normal the baby will be healthy. If he is also a carrier, there is a one in four chance that your fetus may have the condition. Prenatal tests can then be done to find out for certain if your fetus is affected.

Blood group

If you don't already know your blood group it will need to be determined. The groups are O, A, B and AB. O is the most common. Another test is done to find if you are rhesus positive or negative. These tests are done because you may need a blood transfusion at some stage and, before you can have one, your blood group must be known so that blood of the right group can be found. If you are rhesus negative and carry a fetus that is rhesus positive you may develop antibodies to the fetal blood cells – a condition called rhesus haemolytic disease. In the past this could lead to a serious problem for the fetus, but effective preventive treatment is now available (see 'Normal body changes and common problems', page 76).

Rubella

Your immunity to rubella is routinely checked. Rubella used to be called German measles. You were probably immunised as a child but occasionally the immunity weakens. If you are immune, you and your developing baby are protected should you come into contact with someone who has rubella. If you are not immune, you could become infected with rubella and this could be very damaging to your fetus. Therefore, it is very important that you avoid contact with anyone who has the infection. Also, you would normally be given another immunisation after you have had your baby.

Rubella infection in early pregnancy is associated with serious abnormalities in the development of the fetus. These abnormalities affect mainly the eyes, ears and heart, and can result in blindness, deafness and heart defects. The clinical symptoms of rubella can be vague but there is normally a skin rash that lasts 24 hours and you feel unwell for a couple of days. Blood tests can be done to check if you have been infected. If they prove positive and you are in the first couple of months of your pregnancy, most doctors would recommend termination because of the severe congenital defects (present at birth). Immunisation is not recommended in pregnancy.

Hepatitis B and C

Screening for hepatitis B carrier status is routine. You may have had jaundice in the past and this could have been caused by infection from this virus. Sometimes the virus infects your liver with no clinical effects and it may remain in your blood for many years before causing signs of illness.

It is important to know your hepatitis B status so that you can avoid passing infection to your baby. If you are positive your baby will be immunised soon after birth to prevent cross-infection from you. Breast-feeding is best avoided to reduce the risk of transmission to your baby.

Screening for hepatitis C may be indicated if you have a history of substance abuse and in particular intravenous usage. You may be at risk if you have had several sexual partners. Current knowledge suggests that there's no increased risk to the baby if you carry this virus, but you may need treatment.

HIV

You may wish to have your human immunodeficiency virus (HIV) status checked. Most health authorities now offer this routinely, but you may opt out if you so wish. The importance of testing is to reduce the risk of cross-infection from you to your baby if you are positive. This is achieved by giving specific medication to an affected mother and delivering the baby by caesarean section (see page 139). Breast-feeding is best avoided to reduce the risk of transmission to the baby.

The virus can be transmitted when unprotected sex occurs with someone who carries the virus. It is transmitted in blood and seminal fluid (ejaculate) and is more common where there is a history of intravenous drug abuse, prostitution or male homosexuality. HIV attacks the immune system and destroys the body's defences against infection and disease. It can take years for HIV to do enough damage for someone to become ill and develop acquired immune deficiency syndrome (AIDS). Therefore, even if you have no symptoms of AIDS, you may carry the virus. Taking the test will not prevent you from getting life insurance if the result is negative. The Association of British Insurers recommend that applicants should be asked only if they have had a positive HIV test result, not if they have had a test.

Syphilis

Screening for syphilis has been performed for many years. With better hygiene and the use of penicillin for treatment, syphilis is now quite rare. However, it still occurs and can have devastating effects if a baby is infected before birth. If the screen is positive, treatment with a penicillin-based antibiotic is effective.

Glucose and protein in urine

Your urine is tested for glucose at each antenatal visit and you are usually asked to bring a specimen to the clinic. The testing for glucose (a type of sugar) is to check that you are not at risk of developing diabetes during your pregnancy. Diabetes can sometimes develop during pregnancy because your pancreas, which produces insulin, has to work harder. Insulin is required to break down sugar and the reserves of this hormone may be insufficient to meet your pregnancy needs.

In these circumstances, your blood sugars will be high and are likely to spill into your urine. If glucose is found in your urine, you may need further screening for glucose in your blood (a glucose tolerance test). A random blood glucose test may be done later in pregnancy (around 28 weeks) when the demands of your fetus are becoming even greater. This is a screen to check if you have developed diabetes and is more accurate than urine testing.

You can reduce the risk of this happening by modifying your diet to reduce your sugar intake – for example, by cutting out chocolate and sweet drinks. This will reduce your blood glucose levels but, if this is not effective and you show signs of diabetes, you will require insulin.

Your urine is also tested for protein at each antenatal clinic. When protein is present in your urine (proteinuria), it may be the result of kidney problems such as infection or pre-eclampsia (see 'Normal body changes and common problems', page 76). Sometimes it may be caused by contamination from a vaginal discharge.

KEY POINTS

■ A pregnancy test can be done two to three days after a missed period on the early morning urine sample and is 99 per cent accurate

■ The average length of pregnancy is 40 weeks from your last period

■ An early pregnancy scan is done to confirm viability, establish the gestational age and confirm the number of fetuses

■ In any pregnancy a number of blood and urine tests are done – some routine and others selective

Screening for fetal abnormality

Abnormalities in a baby

There is approximately a 1 in 50 chance of abnormality in any baby. Abnormalities range from major ones such as severe heart problems to others that can be treated successfully such as cleft lip. Everyone would prefer a perfect baby but, sadly, life is not like that. However, there are various tests that can screen for specific abnormalities. None of these screening tests is perfect and none guarantees a 100 per cent detection rate.

Blood tests
Alpha-fetoprotein for neural tube defects

This blood test is performed at 16 weeks to screen for the risk of neural tube defects, which are abnormalities that affect the skull bones and brain (anencephaly) or the spine and spinal cord (spina bifida). Anencephaly is a fatal condition.

The spine of our back is made up of a series of bones called vertebrae and these surround the spinal cord. Spina bifida occurs when the vertebrae do not cover the spinal cord completely and there may also be a skin defect so that the membranes around the cord are exposed to infection. The number of bones affected varies as does the amount of spinal cord exposed. However, if an area of the spinal cord is exposed, it can result in paralysis. The defects are more common in the lower back and so the lower limbs are most commonly affected. In the worst cases, control of the bladder and bowel may be affected.

The blood test for alpha-fetoprotein (AFP) is a screening test, not a clear-cut diagnostic test. AFP is normally produced by the liver of the fetus during pregnancy. Therefore, a small amount of AFP in the mother's blood is normal. In late pregnancy, the mother's AFP levels naturally rise, although sometimes AFP levels are high in the earlier stages of pregnancy.

If your level of AFP is abnormally raised, your fetus will have about a 1 in 20 risk of developing a neural

Causes of a raised alpha-fetoprotein

Alpha-fetoprotein (AFP) levels can be checked with a blood test. They may be abnormally raised for various reasons:

- Wrong dates (because the level changes during pregnancy)
- Multiple pregnancy (more than one fetus)
- Threatened miscarriage
- Intrauterine death (death of the fetus)
- Molar pregnancy (a rare condition in which there is a tumour of the placenta)
- Spina bifida, anencephaly
- Some rare abnormalities
- No abnormality but AFP outside normal range

tube defect. If you have a raised level, there are several other possible causes (see box on page 57). You will be sent an appointment to have an ultrasound scan to find out more.

Many hospitals do not perform an AFP test now. As a result of advances in ultrasound imaging, your hospital may prefer to undertake a detailed 18- to 20-week ultrasound scan instead.

Biochemical testing for Down syndrome

Biochemical markers are substances measured in the blood that can alert the obstetrician to the possibility of Down syndrome. Testing is most often done for AFP and human chorionic gonadotrophin (hCG), known as 'the double test' and usually carried out at 15 to 17 weeks. A low AFP and a raised hCG (see 'Confirmation of pregnancy and routine tests', page 37) have been found to be associated with an increased risk of having a baby affected by Down syndrome.

Your age will be computed with the test results to give your actual risk. When your risk is more than 1 in 250, you will usually be seen to discuss if you want a further test, called an amniocentesis (described later in this chapter). Each hospital has a slightly different risk cut-off value.

The double test detects about 60 per cent of affected pregnancies. This means that 40 per cent go undetected. In addition, five per cent of normal unaffected pregnancies will have a falsely positive result on biochemical testing. They are called false positives because in these cases the fetus does not have Down syndrome despite the biochemical test suggesting it was likely.

Another marker called oestriol has been added to the other two (the triple test) but there is doubt whether this adds significant benefit. More recently a further marker called inhibin A has been added to the double and triple tests and has been shown to improve detection by a further 10 per cent (see box below). Most NHS-funded testing uses the double test only. The other tests are available privately.

Much research has been undertaken to see if there are blood tests that can be used to screen earlier in

Detecting Down syndrome

Many tests can be performed to detect Down syndrome in a developing baby. These tests assess the levels or presence of different biochemical markers (substances). Checking for a combination of these markers improves the detection rate.

Age and combination of markers (screening tests)	Detection rate for Down syndrome
Age (> 35 years) without blood testing	30%
Age + AFP	40%
Age + AFP + hCG	60%
Age + AFP + hCG + inhibin A	70%
Age + AFP + hCG + oestriol + inhibin A	75%
Age + PAPP-A + free beta-hCG	60%
Age + nuchal translucency	70%
Age + PAPP-A + free beta-hCG + nuchal translucency	90%

AFP, alpha-fetoprotein; hCG, human chorionic gonadotrophin; PAPP-A, pregnancy-associated plasma protein A.

pregnancy. It appears that the measurement of pregnancy-associated plasma protein A (PAPP-A) and free beta-hCG between 10 and 14 weeks is valuable and can detect around 60 per cent of Down syndrome-affected pregnancies, but this variant of the tests is not in routine use yet.

Ultrasound screening
Measurement of nuchal translucency

Further guidance to the possibility of Down syndrome can come from an ultrasound examination. The skinfold thickness behind the neck of the fetus can be measured (see figure opposite). It is called the nuchal translucency measurement because it is seen on an ultrasound scan as a clear echo-free area of tissue fluid.

An increased, wider, nuchal translucency measurement has been shown to be associated with a number of chromosomal abnormalities, of which the main one is Down syndrome. It has been associated with heart abnormalities but it is also found in fetuses that subsequently turn out to be entirely normal.

When combined with maternal age, nuchal translucency measurements undertaken between 10 and 14 weeks have been shown to detect 70 per cent of fetuses affected with Down syndrome. When nuchal translucency is combined with biochemical screening (as described above), the detection rate has been reported to be as high as 90 per cent.

The measurement can sometimes be difficult to obtain if the fetus is lying in the wrong position. It may also be difficult to see clearly if you are overweight because the ultrasound beam has been weakened on passing through the fat tissue and therefore the image is not so sharp.

Nuchal translucency measurement

This involves using an ultrasound scan to measure the skinfold thickness behind the neck of the fetus. The area measured is seen on the scan as a clear area of tissue fluid. The measurement is most accurate when taken between 7 and 14 weeks of pregnancy.

1. Normal nuchal translucency – 1.3 mm

2. Borderline nuchal translucency – 2.9 mm

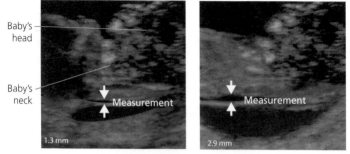

3. Very abnormal nuchal translucency – 6.0 mm

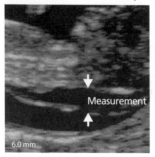

Detailed anatomy scan

This is undertaken between 18 and 22 weeks when all the structures of the fetus can be seen most clearly. Ninety to ninety-five per cent of major structural anomalies will be detected. During the detailed anatomy scan, the sonographer (the technician who carries out the ultrasound scan) will check the anatomical structures in the fetus as listed in the box below.

'Soft markers' are ultrasound markers that have a weak association with chromosomal problems (see box on page 63). They are usually transient findings and are not physical defects. These soft markers can also be found in detailed scans of patients at low risk. In most, the risk of chromosomal problems is less than one per cent and the finding should not cause much unnecessary anxiety. It may be that, when you have a detailed scan, you may not wish the sonographer to

What ultrasound can show

An ultrasound scan taken between weeks 18 and 22 of pregnancy can view the following structures clearly, to check for major structural abnormalities:

- Head shape and size
- Brain structure
- Eye sockets
- Lips
- Spine and covering skin
- Four chambers of the heart
- Major vessels leaving the heart
- Lungs
- Diaphragm
- Stomach
- Kidneys and bladder
- Abdominal wall and cord insertion
- Femur (thigh bone) length
- Arms, legs, hands and feet

look for 'soft' markers. You should be asked whether you want the tests done.

A normal scan is not a guarantee that your baby has no abnormalities because some of these may be undetectable. Cardiac abnormalities are the most difficult to detect and only about one-third of major heart defects are seen in the prenatal scan. Two-thirds of babies with Down syndrome have no major structural abnormality and so the detailed scan will not detect a baby who is affected by the condition.

The only way to be absolutely certain about whether your baby has a chromosomal problem is to grow the cells obtained by an invasive procedure such as amniocentesis or chorionic villus biopsy.

Detailed scans

The sonographer can check for 'soft' markers during the 20-week detailed anatomy ultrasound scan. These soft markers have a weak association with certain chromosomal problems and include:

- Choroid plexus cyst (folds of normal brain tissue containing fluid and appearing cystic)
- Nuchal fold thickening
- Short femur or humerus (leg and arm bones)
- Bright images from part of the bowel
- Bright images from part of the heart
- Dilation of the kidney pelvis (urine-collecting duct)
- Short middle phalanx (bone) of little finger
- Large gap between first and second toes

Invasive tests
Amniocentesis (amnio)

This test is undertaken to determine the number and appearance of the chromosomes (the karyotype) of the cells shed by the fetus, in the amniotic fluid. It is normally performed at 15 weeks when the fluid is plentiful, making the risk of miscarriage less compared with earlier weeks.

A fine needle is passed through the skin of your abdominal wall into the amniotic fluid that surrounds the fetus (see figure opposite). Ultrasound is used to help the doctor guide the needle to the largest, most accessible, pool of fluid. The needle is very fine and the procedure is virtually painless. Twenty millilitres (ml) (an eggcupful) of fluid is taken and sent for analysis.

The fetus is surrounded by about 500 ml of fluid at this time, so only a very small proportion is removed. A small hole has been made in the membranes surrounding the fetus which normally seals immediately. Occasionally in the first 24 hours after the procedure, a leakage of fluid may occur through your vagina. If this persists miscarriage may occur. The procedure is performed under sterile conditions but, on rare occasions, infection can occur and miscarriage results. However, the overall risk of miscarriage is only half to one per cent (1 in 100 to 1 in 200) of all amniocenteses.

The fluid is sent to the genetics laboratory where the cells are grown to check that the chromosomes are normal – a test that has to be done on dividing cells. Laboratories differ in their reporting times – they can vary from two days to three weeks, depending on the methods used. Rarely, in less than one per cent of cases, the test will fail to give a result because of technical problems.

Amniocentesis

An 'amnio' involves passing a fine needle into the amniotic fluid that surrounds the fetus and drawing off a small sample for laboratory testing. Ultrasound is used to guide the needle. The fluid is checked for chromosomal abnormalities.

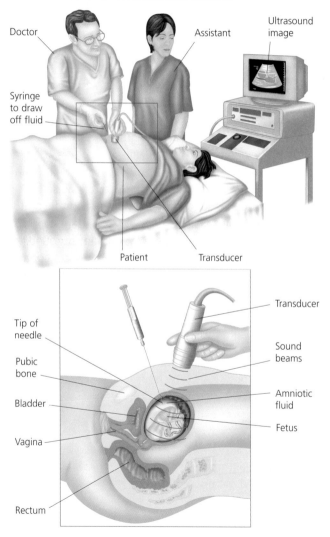

Doctor

Assistant

Ultrasound image

Syringe to draw off fluid

Patient

Transducer

Transducer

Tip of needle

Pubic bone

Bladder

Vagina

Rectum

Sound beams

Amniotic fluid

Fetus

Chorion biopsy or chorionic villus sampling (CVS)

This test is an alternative to amniocentesis for determining whether the chromosomes are normal. It may also be used to diagnose some genetic disorders. It is performed any time after 10 weeks.

The chorion is the early developing placenta and has the same genetic make-up as the fetus. A tiny piece of tissue is taken from the chorion by passing a needle through the abdominal wall and aspirating (gently sucking) a sample up into the needle. A wider needle is used than in amniocentesis but the use of a local anaesthetic makes it virtually painless.

The target site is small and so the procedure is technically more difficult than amniocentesis (see figure). Slight vaginal bleeding is not uncommon afterwards. The miscarriage rate is 1 to 2 per cent (1 in 100 to 1 in 50), which is higher than for amniocentesis but this is partly because it is undertaken at an earlier time when the risk of natural miscarriage is greater.

The cells are cultured (grown) by the genetics laboratory and examined. In 1 per cent (1 in 100) of tests, the laboratory is unable to culture the cells and, in a further 1 per cent (1 in 100), a mixed chromosome pattern (mosaicism) is found which is confined to the chorion and not found in the fetus. The procedure has the advantage of being performed at an earlier time in pregnancy and, for some patients, an early result is welcome, particularly if they are at high risk of having a problem. Laboratories vary in their reporting times – it can be from two days to three weeks.

Chorionic villus sampling (CVS)

The CVS or chorion biopsy removes a tiny piece of tissue from the chorion (early developing placenta) using a needle inserted through the mother's abdominal wall. The procedure is guided by ultrasound. Like an 'amnio', the CVS checks for chromosomal abnormalities.

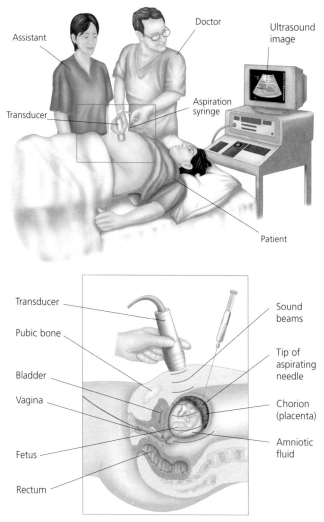

Assistant

Doctor

Ultrasound image

Transducer

Aspiration syringe

Patient

Transducer

Pubic bone

Bladder

Vagina

Fetus

Rectum

Sound beams

Tip of aspirating needle

Chorion (placenta)

Amniotic fluid

Fetal blood sampling

Fetal blood sampling is performed only rarely. It takes a sample of blood from the umbilical cord vein (near where it enters the placenta) under the guidance of ultrasound. The test can check for severe anaemia in the fetus, fetal infections or genetic problems.

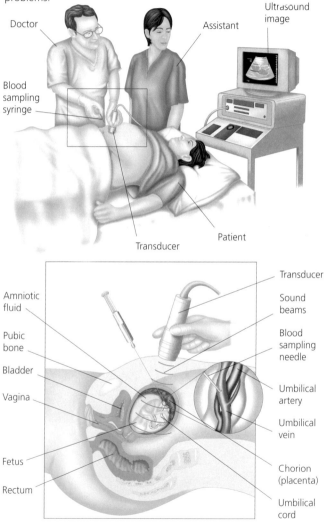

Doctor

Assistant

Ultrasound image

Blood sampling syringe

Transducer

Patient

Amniotic fluid

Pubic bone

Bladder

Vagina

Fetus

Rectum

Transducer

Sound beams

Blood sampling needle

Umbilical artery

Umbilical vein

Chorion (placenta)

Umbilical cord

Fetal blood sampling

This procedure is rarely required and is undertaken only in specialised referral hospitals. It may be undertaken when blood group rhesus antibodies develop (see 'Confirmation of pregnancy and routine tests', page 37) and the fetus is suspected to have severe anaemia. Other reasons that it may be done include diagnosis of fetal infection or genetic problems.

A blood sample is taken from the umbilical cord vein using ultrasound to view the cord at its insertion into the placenta (see figure opposite). The blood can then be sent to a laboratory for testing. Complications may arise and there is a 1 per cent (1 in 100) risk of pregnancy loss as a result of the procedure.

KEY POINTS

- A high AFP (alpha-fetoprotein) level is associated with an increased risk of a neural tube defect

- Biochemical screening for Down syndrome gives a risk factor – there are always false-positive and false-negative results

- Measurement of nuchal translucency should be combined with early biochemical screening – this test is also associated with false-positive and false-negative results

- Detailed anatomy scanning detects 90 to 95 per cent of major abnormalities but is not a guarantee of normality

- Invasive tests are required to provide a reliable diagnosis for chromosome or genetic problems

Antenatal care

Benefits of antenatal care

Antenatal care is the name given to a series of examinations made in the months before a woman goes into labour. The purpose of antenatal care is to screen for problems that are present or likely to develop.

The concept of antenatal care was established in the 1920s when the Ministry of Health devised a formal programme of antenatal visits for at-risk patients who were poor and had had several pregnancies.

This progressively extended to the whole population with 10 to 15 antenatal visits being standard. During the last 10 years it has become obvious that such an intense programme of visits is not necessary in low-risk patients – they probably need only a minimum of four visits. However, some women have substantial social or psychological difficulties and these should be identified and helped as part of antenatal care.

Screening and detection

During the first half of pregnancy, the emphasis is on screening for fetal abnormality and identifying any risk factors in your medical or obstetric history.

During the second half of pregnancy, emphasis is

Minimal care plan for women

Gestation	Content of care	Investigations
8 weeks or first visit to GP/midwife	Obstetric, family and medical history. Height. Weight. Blood pressure. Calculate BMI (see page 3). Calculate EDD. Assess emotional well-being. Refer for appropriate care	Urinalysis (test for sugar and protein). Sickle-cell test (if African–Caribbean or Asian origin). Thalassaemia test (Mediterranean, Asian, Oriental or family history)
12 weeks	Booking ultrasound scan. Review by consultant if problem or patient wishes	
16 weeks	Weight Blood pressure Listen for fetal heart	Urinalysis. Full blood count Blood group. Hepatitis B, rubella, syphilis, HIV. Screen for Down syndrome and spina bifida
20 weeks	Detailed ultrasound scan	
22 weeks	Blood pressure Listen for fetal heart	Urinalysis
28 weeks	Weight. Blood pressure. Oedema (swelling of the ankles, hands, and face). Fundal height measurement. Listen for fetal heart and movements. Give anti-D if rhesus (Rh) negative	Urinalysis Full blood count Blood group Non-fasting blood glucose
32 weeks, first pregnancy only	Blood pressure. Oedema. Fundal height/liquor volume. Fetal heart and movements. Presentation	Urinalysis
34 weeks	Weight (not recommended routinely unless there is an indication). Blood pressure. Oedema. Fundal height/liquor volume. Fetal heart and movements. Presentation. Assess emotional well-being. Give anti-D if Rh negative	Urinalysis
36 weeks, first pregnancy only	Blood pressure. Oedema. Fundal height/liquor volume. Fetal heart and movements. Presentation	Urinalysis
38 weeks	Blood pressure. Oedema. Fundal height/liquor volume. Fetal heart and movements. Presentation	Urinalysis
40 weeks	Blood pressure. Oedema. Fundal height/liquor volume. Fetal heart and movements. Presentation	Urinalysis
41 weeks	Blood pressure. Oedema. Fundal height/liquor volume. Fetal heart and movements. Presentation	Urinalysis

with normal pregnancies

Information and discussion

Personnel

Information leaflets. Exemption certificate FW 8 for dental treatment and prescriptions. Parenthood classes – community/hospital. Smoking, alcohol, diet, posture and exercise, substance misuse, domestic abuse contacts, contact with infections – rubella, etc. Options for care and place of delivery. Roles of GP, community midwife and health visitor and contact numbers. All 16-week blood tests

Midwife/GP

Book detailed scan

Obstetrician/ sonographer

Obtain informed consent for blood tests before taking blood. Discuss detailed ultrasound scan. Health promotion topics as above

Midwife/GP

Sonographer

Mat B1 – employment issues. Information re rhesus negative. Safety and car seatbelts

Midwife/GP

Reminder for parenthood education. Commence discussions on:
• social and domestic arrangements
• place of delivery
• preparation for hospital
• birth plan

Midwife/GP

Midwife/GP

Commence discussions on:
• breast-feeding workshop
• when to contact hospital
• discharge plan
• patterns of postnatal visiting
• support available in postnatal period
• postnatal depression

Midwife/GP

Midwife/GP

Discuss and plan induction of labour (usually 10–13 days after EDD). Vaginal examination and loosening of the membranes if appropriate

Midwife/GP

Midwife/GP

placed on detecting elevated blood pressure and slow growth by the fetus (intrauterine growth restriction). Antepartum haemorrhage (loss of blood from the vagina as a result of bleeding within the uterus) may occur at any time and usually emergency referral is required.

Near your due date, examination of your pregnant abdomen is important to check for malpresentation (when the baby's head is in the wrong position – breech, in which the fetus is positioned head up and bottom down, being the most common problem). Routine blood tests are undertaken at specific intervals as previously described.

Hospital versus community care

If you need specialised care – for example, for diabetes, twins, epilepsy, blood disorders, blood group antibodies or substance misuse – you may be seen at a consultant's clinic. In the clinic, the expertise of the medical and midwifery staff is concentrated to give streamlined care.

If you have no risk factors in your previous medical or obstetric history, your routine antenatal care can take place in the community with your midwife and general practitioner. This appears to be as clinically effective as obstetrician-led care and most women prefer it.

Ideally antenatal care should be woman centred according to personal needs. It should take place locally with access to a specialist if required. Therefore, there should be joint care between community and hospital with a standardised schedule of visits. This results in improved continuity and consistency of care and reduces duplication of care by the hospital and community.

Every maternity hospital establishes its own pattern of care but as women receive their care they can contribute to make it more effective and efficient for all concerned. The box on pages 72–3 gives the outline of a care plan that has been devised for a low-risk patient.

KEY POINTS

- Antenatal care screens for problems that are present or likely to develop

- Antenatal care for patients with no risk factors can take place in the community by midwives and general practitioners

- Patients with specific problems should be seen at a consultant's clinic

Normal body changes and common problems

Hormonal influences

Occasionally pregnancy is associated with symptoms and signs that are unpleasant and may make you feel unwell. They are the result of the hormonal influences of pregnancy and the physical changes that occur in your body. If you were not pregnant your doctor would be concerned that you had a serious illness. It is not unknown for patients who deny that they are pregnant to be investigated for serious illness.

There are no cures for these normal symptoms but only simple remedies that may help. It is important to understand that they will not harm you and that most will go away after pregnancy.

Normal body changes of pregnancy

The characteristic first symptoms of pregnancy are nausea, urinary frequency and breast tenderness. Your breasts will begin to feel heavy in the early months of pregnancy as a result of the increase in glandular activity and you will find that your bust size will increase. Your nipples will also darken (and will do so again in later pregnancies) and, by four months, you may find that clear fluid is being secreted. This is an early form of breast milk called colostrum.

If you have fair skin, you will find that your skin may darken during pregnancy and if you are exposed to the sun you will tan more easily. When you look in the mirror, you will be darker under the eyes and this darkness may extend across your cheeks. This is called chloasma, the mask of pregnancy. A dark line will also be seen down the middle of your waist, more so beneath your navel. This is called the linea nigra (Latin for 'black line'). All these changes in pigmentation are caused by hormones secreted by the pituitary gland.

You may not notice any enlargement of your waist until four months have passed. If you are very thin and you press your hand in the lower part of your abdomen, you may feel your pregnant uterus arising from the pelvis after 12 weeks. It is normally easily felt after 16 weeks. As your pregnancy increases in size, your overlying skin will be stretched. Often, thin red stretch marks will appear on your abdomen and sometimes on your breasts. These are called striae gravidarum and they fade after pregnancy to remain as white marks called striae albicantes and never disappear completely.

Fetal movements

As the uterus increases in size, you will begin to feel your fetus moving. Exactly when this happens varies quite markedly. The first movements feel as if you have butterflies in your stomach, a fluttering sensation. In your first pregnancy, this usually happens between 18 and 22 weeks whereas, in subsequent pregnancies, it tends to be earlier at 16 to 20 weeks. The movements become more pronounced as your pregnancy proceeds – and in later pregnancy you may have difficulty having a peaceful night's sleep! Your perception of fetal movements will vary from pregnancy to pregnancy and not all the movements of your baby are felt. In the last three months of pregnancy at least 10 movements should be felt from 9am to 9pm. If your mind is occupied with other activities, you are less likely to be aware of movements. Later in pregnancy you may be asked to count the number of movements in a period of time as a low-tech, safe way of confirming the health of the fetus.

Braxton Hicks contractions

As your pregnancy nears its end you may find that your uterus hardens for 20 to 40 seconds every now and again. These are contractions of the muscle of your uterus wall and are called Braxton Hicks contractions. They can sometimes feel so strong that you may think labour is starting and it can be difficult to distinguish true from false labour. Usually labour is established when there are three to five good, regular, strong contractions in 10 minutes, each contraction lasting 40 to 60 seconds (see 'Labour and delivery', page 109).

Common pregnancy-related problems
Heartburn

This is a common symptom, more frequent in late pregnancy as a result of increasing levels of your hormones and the increasing size of your pregnancy delaying the emptying of your stomach. This leads to your stomach acids refluxing (overflowing) into the lower part of your oesophagus (the narrow elastic tube connecting your mouth and stomach). The acid reflux causes irritation (see figure on page 80).

The symptom is a feeling of burning behind your breast bone in the lower central chest area. As it is caused by overflow of stomach acids, measures can be taken to reduce the discomfort.

Certain foods are more commonly associated with heartburn and you will quickly realise which ones affect you. Generally, those foods that trigger excess stomach acids will cause heartburn: fatty or spicy foods and also strong tea. In addition, a large meal will require excess stomach acids for digestion and so it makes sense to have frequent small meals rather than fewer large ones.

When you are sitting or standing, the acids naturally drain from your stomach. If you are stooping or lying down, reflux of acid into your oesophagus is more likely to occur. Heartburn can be reduced if you avoid eating late in the evening or if you prop yourself up on pillows so that you are not lying flat in bed.

When you get heartburn, you can try drinking some water to dilute the stomach acid. If this does not help, you can safely take some simple medications to neutralise the acid. These are called antacids and the most commonly used is Gaviscon. If your symptoms are severe and persistent, you may require a prescription from your doctor for an acid-suppressing drug, such as cimetidine or ranitidine. The medicines recommended by your doctor have all been used for many years by thousands of women without any evidence of harm to the baby.

Heartburn

Gastro-oesophageal reflux (heartburn) occurs when the stomach contents leak into the oesophagus. Medication often contains an antacid to reduce the acidity of the stomach contents and alginate, which floats on the stomach contents; if reflux occurs the alginate soothes the lining of the oesophagus.

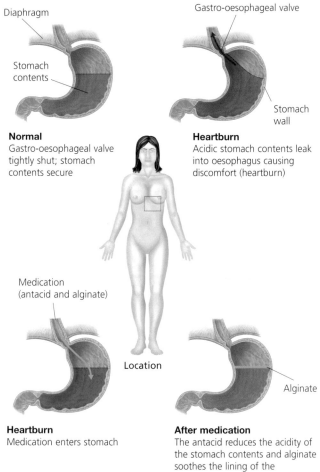

Diaphragm

Stomach contents

Normal
Gastro-oesophageal valve tightly shut; stomach contents secure

Gastro-oesophageal valve

Stomach wall

Heartburn
Acidic stomach contents leak into oesophagus causing discomfort (heartburn)

Location

Medication (antacid and alginate)

Heartburn
Medication enters stomach

Alginate

After medication
The antacid reduces the acidity of the stomach contents and alginate soothes the lining of the oesophagus

Nausea and vomiting

Most women experience nausea in early pregnancy and in some it is combined with vomiting. It does not usually last beyond the first three months of pregnancy. Rarely, episodes may be prolonged with excessive vomiting (hyperemesis) when admission to hospital is required.

The symptoms can occur any time of day even though it is commonly called 'morning sickness'. There are some simple measures that can be taken to help:

- You will normally find that certain things trigger the feeling of nausea and vomiting. If it is the sight or smell of certain foods, you can avoid them

- It is better to take frequent small snacks rather than big meals

- Bland, uncomplicated foods are easier to hold down such as bananas, dried fruit, potatoes, rice or biscuits

- Sitting still and having a rest will also help, for some women, if you can arrange it

- There is some evidence to suggest that acupuncture at the wrist will help and some find that wrist bands used for travel sickness help.

Medication is best avoided in the first three months of pregnancy but sometimes this is required for excessive nausea and vomiting. Your doctor may prescribe an antihistamine or antiemetic. Like the antacids mentioned above these drugs have been used in thousands of pregnant women and are generally considered safe. They are likely to make you feel drowsy and occasionally you can get double vision. If you have hyperemesis (excessive and prolonged vomiting), you will have to be admitted to hospital for intravenous fluid replacement and the administration of medication. In extreme cases, steroids are sometimes required.

Constipation

This is more common as pregnancy advances. It is caused by two factors:

1. The pregnancy hormone progesterone which causes muscle relaxation so that the muscular contractions of the bowel are less forceful.

2. The physical effect of the growing fetus compressing the large bowel in the pelvis.

The infrequent passage of hard stools can result in abdominal pains as a result of the build-up of impacted faeces and so it is important to take measures to reduce constipation.

Diet, fluid intake and exercise affect the movement of your bowels. Constipation can be reduced by eating more fibre and so increasing the bulk of your diet. Fibre is found in cereals, fruit and vegetables. If you eat more fibre you will also need to drink more water – so take a glass of water with food and between meals. Many women find that constipation is less of a problem if they take gentle exercise, such as going for a short walk or a swim. You can do this as often as you like so long as you continue to enjoy the exercise.

If these simple measures fail, you should try taking some bran. If this is not enough, you can try laxatives such as cellulose bulking agents and stool softeners. Irritant laxatives such as castor oil and bisacodyl should be avoided because they may bring on premature labour but, if the constipation is very troublesome, your doctor may agree that they may be necessary. Enemas are best avoided for the same reason.

Haemorrhoids (piles)

There is a network of veins in your lower rectum, just inside your anus. These can enlarge and protrude so that you will feel them as small lumps at your anus. These are haemorrhoids or piles (see figure below). They may cause itching and pain and may bleed on passing a bowel motion. The increasing pressure of the weight of your pregnancy causes these veins to increase in size, dilate and protrude. They are difficult to avoid.

Anything that increases the pressure within your abdomen will increase the tendency for haemorrhoids. Using a bidet or shower hose after a bowel motion will

Haemorrhoids (piles)

There is a network of veins just inside the anus (back passage). The pressure and weight of pregnancy can cause these veins to enlarge and protrude, forming haemorrhoids or piles. This can cause itching and pain.

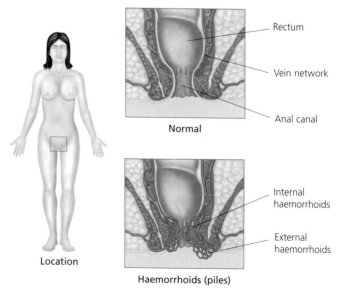

Location

Normal

Rectum

Vein network

Anal canal

Internal haemorrhoids

External haemorrhoids

Haemorrhoids (piles)

keep the area clean and reduce irritation from wiping. Resting with your legs up and avoiding constipation will help. If your haemorrhoids are sore, sitting on crushed ice in a plastic bag will give some relief. Soothing creams and suppositories (solid medication inserted into the anus where it dissolves) can be bought over the pharmacy counter. Anusol is the most commonly used. Usually the piles go away after delivery.

Backache and symphyseal pain

Your body has to alter its posture to carry the pregnancy. The burden of weight is in your lower abdomen and so the curvature of your lower back changes. The fixed joints in your pelvis are the sacroiliac and symphysis pubis – these soften during pregnancy and become more flexible to allow your baby to pass through the pelvis more easily at birth. There is also increasing weight and pressure on your symphysis pubis. So it is not surprising that backache and pain over the pubic symphysis (symphyseal pain) are common in later pregnancy.

The pain should go away once you've had your baby. Wearing comfortable shoes is important and you will usually find that flat ones without a heel are best. Sit on chairs with good back support and avoid heavy lifting. Lying on your side with your knees bent may help. A pelvic brace will give additional support to your symphysis pubic joint and your midwife can help arrange this.

Swelling of hands and feet (oedema)

During the last 10 weeks of pregnancy, your body tends to retain water and you will initially be aware of this in your hands when you find difficulty fitting your rings. You may also find that your shoes are tighter and your ankles are swelling. These are normal features of most pregnancies.

Sometimes the swelling in your hands can become so much that you experience numbness and pins and needles in your fingers – usually your thumb and first and second fingers. The sensation is worst in the morning because fluid is redistributed while you are lying in bed. The extra fluid presses on and irritates your median nerve where it passes in a tissue tunnel between the bones of your wrist. This group of symptoms is called carpal tunnel syndrome. If the symptoms are severe, relief can be obtained by wearing a splint to reduce wrist movement. More generalised swelling involving the face may also be an early sign of pre-eclampsia when your blood pressure will also be increased (see page 98).

Varicose veins

Each leg has two large veins on the surface, just under the skin. One is in the inner aspect of the leg and is called the long saphenous vein. The other is on the outside of the lower leg and is called the short saphenous vein (see figure on page 86). When standing, the blood in these veins is under increased pressure as a result of the force of gravity acting on the blood in the circulation.

During late pregnancy, the pressure is greater because your increased weight acts to increase the pressure in the veins; also because of lower activity the flow of blood back to the heart from your legs is slowed. Your leg veins may become distended and tortuous. Sometimes this extends to involve the veins on your vulva and these are seen as vulval varicosities. They will never burst but there may be a sensation of

Formation of varicose veins

In late pregnancy, when standing, the blood in the veins of the legs is under increased pressure. As a result the leg veins may become varicose, distended and tortuous.

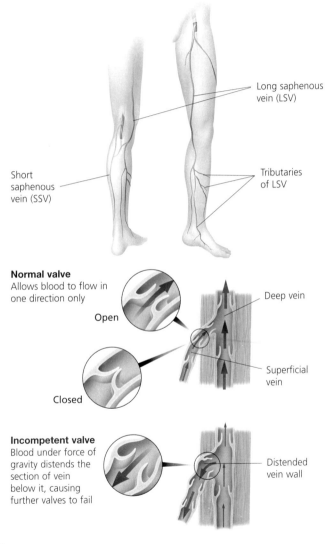

Long saphenous vein (LSV)

Tributaries of LSV

Short saphenous vein (SSV)

Normal valve
Allows blood to flow in one direction only

Open

Closed

Deep vein

Superficial vein

Incompetent valve
Blood under force of gravity distends the section of vein below it, causing further valves to fail

Distended vein wall

heaviness, throbbing, tingling or occasionally pain in your affected veins.

The treatment is to avoid standing for long periods. If standing cannot be avoided it is helpful to keep moving your legs to avoid the blood pooling in your veins under pressure and putting excessive pressure on the vein walls. Elastic stockings or tights give support and reduce the distension in your veins. Resting with your legs up will also help.

Leg cramps

Cramps are involuntary contractions of the muscles causing pain and difficulty using the affected limb, usually a leg. These sometimes occur in late pregnancy, but the cause is unknown. The cramp takes the form of painful hardness in the affected muscle and this may often waken you at night. The best treatment is to massage the affected muscle vigorously. The use of calcium or salt tablets has not proved to be of benefit.

Vaginal discharge

The secretory glands of the cervix are more active during pregnancy and these secretions naturally cause more vaginal discharge than usual. No measures are required to reduce or change the nature of this normal discharge.

The discharge should not be itchy or offensive. Occasionally, it may be itchy and this is usually as a result of thrush (a candidal infection) which is more common in pregnancy. It is caused by a fungus (*Candida*) and is easily treated with an imidazole pessary prescribed by your doctor.

If the discharge has an offensive odour, it is often a bacterial or trichomonas infection of the vagina. A

The calf muscle and compression stockings

The contraction of muscles compressing veins helps push blood up through the leg veins back to the heart. The valves allow the blood to flow towards the heart only.

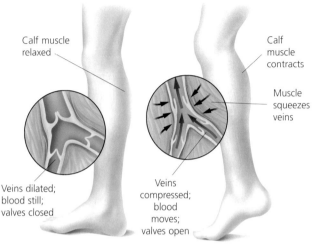

Calf muscle relaxed

Calf muscle contracts

Muscle squeezes veins

Veins dilated; blood still; valves closed

Veins compressed; blood moves; valves open

Compression narrows the superficial leg veins by squeezing them. This results in a smaller volume of blood in the veins and helps the flow in the deep veins.

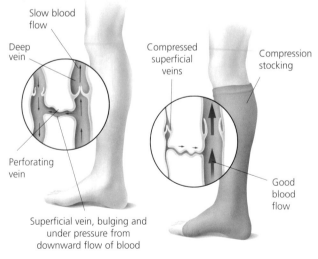

Slow blood flow

Deep vein

Compressed superficial veins

Compression stocking

Perforating vein

Good blood flow

Superficial vein, bulging and under pressure from downward flow of blood

vaginal swab may be taken and a course of metronidazole tablets is usually an effective treatment. As with all medications, it is better to avoid them in the first three months of pregnancy unless completely necessary.

Most vaginal infections are completely harmless to your baby. However, some may be passed to your baby if left untreated – group B streptococci, chlamydia infection and gonococci. It has not been found effective to screen all pregnant patients for vaginal organisms.

Group B streptococci are present in 10 to 15 per cent of patients as a normal organism but in a few rare instances it may take the opportunity to infect the baby (and cause serious blood poisoning, especially if the baby is pre-term [before 37 weeks] or low birthweight). This rarely happens but, if you were found to have the organism, it would be recommended that you have antibiotics during labour.

Chlamydia infection and gonococci can cause an eye infection in the newborn. A sticky eye in your baby may be a sign of such infection and swabs would be taken to check this. If infection is found to be present, your baby would require treatment with antibiotics and you would need treatment too.

Tiredness

With all these possible symptoms it is not surprising that tiredness is a feature of pregnancy. It tends to predominate in early pregnancy when nausea is a problem and then in late pregnancy when you are uncomfortable and the baby is moving more. It is common to have disturbed sleep. You may have to alter your work schedule such that you can have a nap during the day.

KEY POINTS

- Nausea, urinary frequency and breast tenderness are common in the first few months of pregnancy

- Skin changes include darkening around the eyes, linea nigra and striae

- Swelling of the hands and feet, heartburn, constipation, haemorrhoids and varicose veins are common in late pregnancy

- Backache and pain in the symphysis pubis normally resolve soon after delivery

- Excessive non-offensive vaginal discharge is normal

- It is best to avoid medication during the first three months of pregnancy but sometimes this may be necessary for severe symptoms

Complications

Vaginal bleeding

Vaginal bleeding is a common complication in pregnancy. When it occurs before 24 weeks the fetus is not considered viable (it is incapable of survival outside the uterus) and the bleeding is referred to as a 'threatened miscarriage'. This doesn't necessarily mean that miscarriage will occur.

If vaginal bleeding happens after 24 weeks, it is called an antepartum haemorrhage. It is not normal to

Causes of antepartum haemorrhage

When vaginal bleeding occurs after 24 weeks of pregnancy, this is called an antepartum haemorrhage:

- Placenta praevia (misplaced placenta)
- Abruption (bleeding behind the placenta)
- Vasa praevia (blood vessels overlying the presenting part – the baby's head or buttocks – whichever is in position to come out first)
- Local cause (cervical polyp – a small harmless growth – or a cervical cancer or a fungus infection – see 'Vaginal discharge', page 87)
- Unknown or indeterminate

have vaginal bleeding at this stage of the pregnancy and it must always be investigated to find a possible cause (see box on page 91). In most instances, the bleeding is slight and a cause is never found. When this happens, it is thought to be caused by bleeding from the veins at the edge of the placenta. This does not harm the fetus or mother.

However, major haemorrhage (profuse bleeding) can occur with serious consequences for the mother and fetus. There are two main causes of serious haemorrhage: placenta praevia (a misplaced placenta) and abruption (bleeding behind the placenta).

Placenta praevia

Placenta praevia occurs when the placenta lies low in the uterus below the presenting part – head or buttocks. This means that the birth canal is obstructed to a varying degree by the placenta. If the placenta starts to peel off the uterus, there will be painless bleeding. There are various degrees of placenta praevia and the use of ultrasound scanning helps to make this diagnosis (see figure opposite).

Major placenta praevia is the most serious problem in that it is associated with recurring, painless bleeding and, ultimately, the baby will have to be delivered by caesarean section. If you develop this problem, it is likely that you will have to stay in hospital so that you can be delivered as an emergency should heavy bleeding occur. The bleeding does not harm the development of your baby but it does carry a risk for your health. Continual recurrent bleeding will make you anaemic and, if the bleeding is profuse, blood transfusion will

Placenta praevia

In placenta praevia, the placenta lies too low down in the uterus, which can obstruct the birth canal to a varying degree.

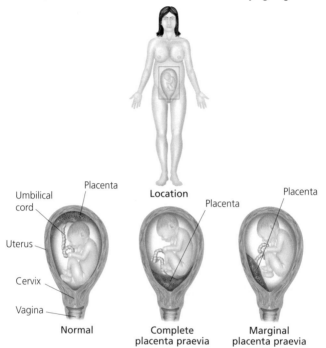

Location

Umbilical cord
Placenta
Placenta
Placenta
Uterus
Cervix
Vagina

Normal
Complete placenta praevia
Marginal placenta praevia

be necessary. Sometimes the bleeding is only slight and delivery will normally be planned for 38 weeks by caesarean section.

Abruption

Abruption (abruptio placentae) occurs when there is bleeding (haemorrhage) behind the placenta (see figure on page 94). This may be contained behind the placenta and so vaginal bleeding will not always occur. If the haemorrhage is large, it will be painful and the uterus becomes hard and tender.

Placental abruption

Abruption occurs when there is bleeding (haemorrhage) behind the placenta. A revealed abruption causes vaginal bleeding whereas a concealed abruption retains the blood within the uterus.

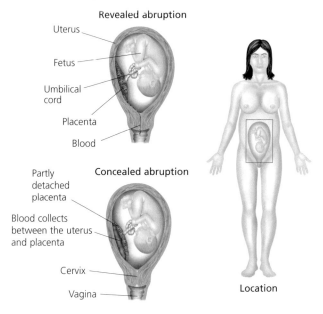

Revealed abruption

Uterus

Fetus

Umbilical cord

Placenta

Blood

Concealed abruption

Partly detached placenta

Blood collects between the uterus and placenta

Cervix

Vagina

Location

When a serious abruption develops, the placenta becomes separated from the uterus, reducing the exchange of oxygen and nutrients to the fetus. There are varying degrees of the problem but, when the placenta is completely detached, the oxygen supply to the fetus is cut off and it can survive only for a few minutes. When abruption is diagnosed and the fetus is still alive, delivery is undertaken as quickly as possible, usually by emergency caesarean section. Even then, the baby may be lost.

Investigation of bleeding

If you have vaginal bleeding after 24 weeks, you must have a check-up. The extent of the investigations will depend on how much bleeding you have but you will need examination and investigations to exclude a serious cause for the bleeding.

Your vagina will be examined using a speculum (an instrument to help view the vagina and cervix). If the

Investigating vaginal bleeding

If you have vaginal bleeding after 24 weeks, you must have a check-up. Your vagina will be examined using a speculum to help view the vagina and cervix and check for any abnormal vaginal discharge.

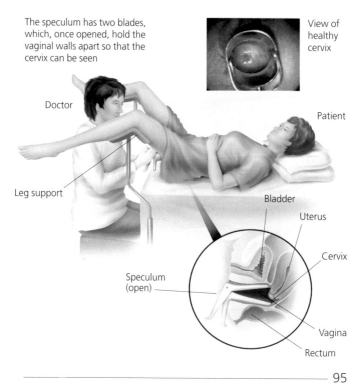

The speculum has two blades, which, once opened, hold the vaginal walls apart so that the cervix can be seen

View of healthy cervix

Doctor

Patient

Leg support

Bladder

Uterus

Cervix

Speculum (open)

Vagina

Rectum

bleeding has occurred after sex, it is likely that it has come from your cervix or vagina and is not serious. This is why it is important to have a vaginal speculum examination to check that your cervix appears normal and that there is no abnormal vaginal discharge. During pregnancy, the cervix becomes very vascular and the glandular elements of the inner cervix become exposed. This is called cervical ectopy (or erosion) and bleeding may easily occur on contact. Rarely a cancer of the cervix may be found in pregnancy.

You will also have an ultrasound examination to locate the site of the placenta and to look for any blood clot behind it. A tracing of the fetal heart rate may also be undertaken and you may need to be admitted into hospital until the bleeding is seen to settle.

Pre-term labour

The onset of labour before 37 completed weeks is called pre-term labour. In most cases there is no obvious reason why the early onset of labour occurs but, in some, there is a reason and the reasons are listed in the box opposite.

A diagnosis of pre-term labour can be difficult to make in the early stages and often patients are admitted in false pre-term labour. This usually presents as a bout of uterine contractions that seem like the real thing but, if the cervix does not shorten or dilate, pre-term labour will not occur.

If you are concerned that you may be in labour pre-term, it is better to be checked out because a pre-term baby will require special care. The amount of care relates closely to the number of weeks of pregnancy rather than the birthweight. Respiratory distress syndrome (difficulty breathing owing to immaturity of

Reasons for pre-term labour

If you have had a pre-term delivery, there is a slightly higher chance that it may happen again. It may be possible to reduce the risk if the cause can be found. The main causes are:

- Multiple pregnancy (more than one fetus)
- Polyhydramnios (too much fluid in the uterus)
- Physical abnormality of uterus such as a double cavity
- Cervical incompetence (cervix dilates too readily)
- Infection (listeriosis, toxoplasmosis)
- Antepartum haemorrhage (see page 91)
- Trauma, for example, from road accident
- Maternal illness such as diabetes
- Unknown

the lungs) is one of the main complications for a pre-term baby, particularly if born before 35 weeks. The severity of this complication can be reduced if the mother is given a 24-hour course of steroid injections before the birth. This helps to mature the fetal lungs. In some instances, the doctors may try to suppress the contractions with intravenous medication so that the course of steroids can be given.

Premature rupture of the membranes

Pre-term, premature rupture of the membranes may happen several weeks before the expected onset of labour. Once the membranes have ruptured, you will require daily checks to make sure there is no evidence of infection. If infection does set in, you will need to be delivered without delay.

There is usually no obvious reason why the membranes rupture prematurely but there does appear to be an association with the growth of certain types of bacteria in the vagina. This relationship is difficult to establish clearly because the vagina is not sterile and always harbours bacteria. It is known that certain bacteria produce enzymes that can break down the amniotic membrane tissue. However, the use of antibiotics to eradicate these bacteria has not been successful in preventing the recurrence of pre-term labour in a later pregnancy.

Cervical incompetence

In a small percentage of cases the cervix is found to be weak and dilates with little in the way of uterine contractions. This is called cervical incompetence and is normally associated with delivery in the second three months. When this is thought to be the reason for pre-term labour, a stitch may be inserted into your cervix to strengthen it and reduce the risk of recurrence.

Pregnancy-induced high blood pressure or pre-eclampsia

This is one of the most common complications of pregnancy affecting 5 to 10 per cent of all pregnant women after 24 weeks' gestation. Its features include raised blood pressure, fluid retention causing swelling of the legs and gain in weight, and protein in the urine. Without treatment it may cause serious disease in both mother and baby.

If protein is found in the urine it indicates leakage through the normal kidney filters (proteinuria) and the disorder is called proteinuric pre-eclampsia. Normally there are no symptoms but occasionally it may be accompanied by headache, flashing lights and pain in the upper abdomen; there may also be visible oedema (swelling) of the legs and face. In severe cases, it may lead to convulsions called eclamptic fits and may be life threatening to the mother. The symptoms disappear after delivery and early delivery is the only cure when it is severe.

The time in pregnancy when this complication develops and its severity both vary. The severity is assessed from your blood pressure, the amount of protein in your urine and the results of blood tests (see box on page 100).

Checking for pre-eclampsia
Blood pressure
Two measurements are taken when your blood pressure is recorded. The higher number is the systolic pressure and the lower the diastolic pressure. The diastolic readings are more important for assessing pregnancy-induced hypertension (PIH). A diastolic pressure of more than 90 on two occasions, four hours apart, is in keeping with PIH. When the diastolic is above 100 it is of more concern and oral medication may be given to lower the pressure. When the diastolic is more than 110, it is considered serious and you are usually given intravenous medication to lower your blood pressure and your baby is delivered.

Protein in the urine
The appearance of protein in your urine is of concern if you also have high blood pressure. Protein in the urine is recorded using '+' signs. Persistent recordings of ++, +++, ++++ are seen if you have significant proteinuria and this shows that protein is leaking from your kidneys into your urine. The cause of the kidney damage is unclear, but it is usually only temporary and like other features of pre-eclampsia it clears up once the baby has been

delivered. Nevertheless, when tests persistently show protein in the urine, this indicates that your pre-eclampsia is moderate to severe and delivery will be considered depending on how advanced the pregnancy is and blood test results.

Blood tests

The blood tests will check how many platelets you have in your blood (platelets are vital for stopping bleeding) and will measure the urate level, a good guide to the condition of your kidneys. Liver function tests will assess the liver. If your urate is high, platelets low and liver function tests abnormal, this indicates that your pre-eclampsia is severe and that your baby should be delivered.

Checks for pre-eclampsia

Pregnancy-induced hypertension (PIH or pre-eclampsia) can be diagnosed from the following checks.

1. **Blood pressure**
   A diastolic pressure of more than 90 on two occasions, 4 hours apart, is a sign of PIH. When the diastolic pressure is above 100, oral medication may be required. When the diastolic pressure is over 110, this is considered serious and intravenous medication is usually given.

2. **Protein in the urine**
   This is of concern if the blood pressure is high as well. Persistent high levels (recorded as ++, +++ or ++++) indicate the severity of the pre-eclampsia.

3. **Blood tests**
   If urate levels are high, platelets are low and liver function tests are abnormal, the pre-eclampsia is severe and the baby needs to be delivered.

If you are found to have pre-eclampsia, your fetus will be assessed because placental blood flow is often reduced and intrauterine growth is restricted. If there is evidence that the fetus is at risk of immediate damage, delivery will be required. If severe pre-eclampsia develops at an early gestation (between 24 and 26 weeks), the chances of survival for your baby are less good. Your obstetrician would have to balance the risks to you against the risks for your baby. In extreme (and very rare) circumstances the pregnancy may need to be terminated to save the mother's life.

Intrauterine growth restriction

Some fetuses grow more slowly than would be expected and may be at risk of an adverse outcome. In most cases the causes of intrauterine growth restriction (IUGR) are unknown. If IUGR is detected in early pregnancy, it may be the result of a chromosomal disorder, infection or genetic predisposition. If it occurs later, it is usually caused by loss of growth support from the placenta. This can happen with pre-eclampsia, diabetes or other maternal disorders including smoking and other lifestyle factors such as drug abuse.

An important part of antenatal care is for the midwife or the doctor to measure the fundal height of the uterus (see figure on page 102) with a tape measure. This is to look for signs of suspected IUGR, when it will usually be followed by an ultrasound scan to assess the growth of the fetus and the amniotic fluid volume. The most accurate way of assessing the growth of the fetus is to measure the abdominal circumference. The measurement is plotted on centile charts, which provide an instant verdict on whether

Measuring the baby's growth

During pregnancy, the doctor or midwife measures the fundal height of the uterus with a tape measure. This involves measuring the distance from the top of the uterus to the top of the pubic bone.

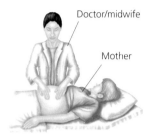
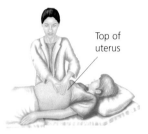

Doctor/midwife

Mother

Top of uterus

1. Mother lies flat on a bed with empty bladder

2. Doctor locates the top of the uterus

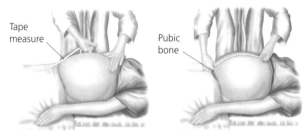

Tape measure

Pubic bone

3. Doctor secures tape measure to top of uterus

4. Doctor measures to the top of the pubic bone

growth is in line with data from large numbers of healthy babies (see figure opposite) and may be repeated every two weeks.

If the growth seems poor and the amniotic fluid is reduced, the blood flow in the umbilical artery may be assessed using an ultrasound machine. The obstetrician has to judge when it is better to deliver the baby rather than leaving it inside to become more mature.

Ultrasound growth chart

An ultrasound scan can be performed to check the growth of the fetus. The measurements can be plotted on a chart to check that the growth is in line with that of large numbers of healthy babies at a similar age.

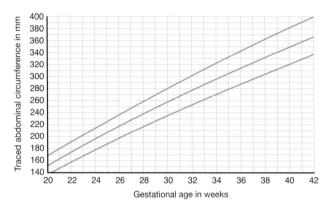

Urinary tract infection

When you are pregnant, you are prone to urinary infections because urine collects in your ureters (two tubes that carry urine from the kidney to the bladder). There are two reasons for this. First, the pregnancy hormone progesterone causes the smooth muscle of the ureter to relax and, second, the ureters are compressed by the pregnant uterus as they cross the brim of the pelvis.

This static urine may become infected and cause inflammation of the ureters and kidneys (pyelonephritis). This is more common on the right side. Sometimes the bladder becomes inflamed (cystitis).

The symptoms of a urinary infection vary, depending on which parts of the urinary tract are affected and how severe the infection is. Around five per cent of pregnant women have a large number of bacteria in their urine but have no symptoms. This is called asymptomatic bacteriuria. It is known that such patients have a higher risk of developing a urinary infection later in pregnancy, but treatment is not usually given until symptoms develop. The main symptoms are pain when you pass urine, a need to empty the bladder at frequent intervals, and in severe cases pain in the back or low in the abdomen and a fever. Treatment with antibiotics will usually clear up the symptoms.

Other infections

Other infections are uncommon. There are a few infections that cause a flu-like illness in adults and if they spread to the fetus may cause a miscarriage or birth defects. These are parvovirus, cytomegalovirus, listeriosis and toxoplasmosis. These infections are rare and so a universal screening policy is not justified. You should, however, be aware of them and avoid contact if possible.

Parvovirus

Parvovirus causes 'slapped cheek' disease, which is a fever with red cheeks. Other symptoms may include arthritis. If a child has this, avoid contact and, if you have symptoms yourself, talk to your doctor about the need for blood tests, because in the developing fetus the virus may slow the production of red blood cells by the bone marrow.

Cytomegalovirus

Cytomegalovirus causes only a mild flu-like illness in adults, but if it spreads to the fetus it may cause a miscarriage or deafness. Later in pregnancy it may cause problems at birth such as jaundice.

Listeriosis
The risk of contracting listeriosis can be reduced by avoiding goats' milk and soft or unpasteurised cheeses. Again the infection may cause a miscarriage or the newborn baby may have an infection such as meningitis.

Toxoplasmosis
Toxoplasmosis is a parasitic infection that may damage the retina at the back of the eye. To avoid the infection do not handle raw or uncooked meats and use gloves if cleaning a cat's litter tray.

Chickenpox
Chickenpox tends to cause more serious symptoms in the pregnant woman rather than the fetus.

Genital herpes
Genital herpes is of concern if blisters are present around the time of delivery. You should inform your obstetrician if you think you might be infected because of the risk to the baby of developing generalised herpes, which may cause a life-threatening infective illness.

Rhesus disease
This condition occurs when a mother develops antibodies to the red blood cells of her fetus, resulting in the baby becoming anaemic (deficient in red blood cells). Without treatment the problem becomes worse and occurs earlier with each pregnancy.

When you have your blood group tested you will be told that it is A, B, AB or O, and that you are either rhesus (Rh) positive (85 per cent of Europeans) or negative (the other 15 per cent). You will possibly have problems if you are Rh negative and your partner is Rh positive.

The rhesus factor is named after the type of monkey (rhesus) in which it was first identified. When a mother who is Rh negative carries a baby who is Rh positive the baby's red cells will stimulate the mother to form antibodies called anti-D; fetal blood enters her bloodstream to trigger the reaction.

Fetal cells enter into the maternal circulation most commonly at delivery but may also do so during pregnancy, if the mother has a 'sensitising event' – a miscarriage, a termination of pregnancy, a procedure such as amniocentesis or external cephalic version (turning a breech baby).

Leakage of blood to the mother at birth does not affect the newly born fetus, but the mother's immune system becomes sensitised and in the next pregnancy the antibody response occurs earlier and more rapidly. The maternal antibodies cross the placenta into the fetal circulation. The antibodies attach to the fetal red blood cells and the cells break down, causing the fetus to become anaemic. This can be so severe that the fetus may need to be transfused while still in the uterus, otherwise death from anaemia would occur.

Preventing rhesus disease

Fortunately, this problem (known as rhesus disease) has almost been eliminated in the developed world because of the use of anti-D immunoglobulin (anti-D). If you are Rh negative you will be given an injection of this after delivery or after a sensitising event during pregnancy (see above).

The immunoglobulin contains antibodies, which attach to any fetal red blood cells that may be in your circulation. The injection usually prevents your immune system becoming sensitised by destroying the fetal red blood cells in the mother's bloodstream.

The time of greatest risk of the fetal blood entering your bloodstream is during labour and at delivery. After delivery your baby's blood group is checked and, if it is Rh positive (and you are Rh negative) you will be given an anti-D injection.

Your blood will also be tested because sometimes it can have a lot of fetal cells in it. If this is so, you will be given more than one injection of anti-D. If your baby is Rh negative, an injection is not necessary.

There is now evidence to show that, by giving anti-D to mothers who are Rh negative at approximately 28 and 34 weeks, the risk of developing antibodies is reduced from 15 per 1,000 cases to 2 per 1,000. Anti-D is also given to Rh-negative patients if they have a sensitising event (see above).

Anti-D injections are made from donated blood that is screened for viral infections, including HIV. It is made from plasma from the USA to avoid the tiny risk of new variant Creutzfeldt–Jakob disease or CJD (bovine spongiform encephalopathy [BSE] or mad cow disease). Anti-D has been used in pregnancy for over 30 years and many millions of injections have been given without any known problems, so it appears to be without risk.

KEY POINTS

- In most cases of antepartum haemorrhage (bleeding from the vagina), no cause is found but placenta praevia, abruption or a local anatomical cause must be excluded

- Respiratory distress is one of the main complications suffered by a pre-term infant

- Pregnancy-induced high blood pressure is more serious when there is proteinuria (protein in the urine) or an abnormal blood test result

- When intrauterine growth restriction develops, the clinical decision has to be made about whether it is safer to deliver the fetus or continue the pregnancy

- Infections of the urinary tract are more common than other infections in pregnancy

- The use of anti-D has almost eliminated rhesus disease in the developed world

Labour and delivery

The onset of labour

The onset of labour is the exciting event that means
your baby will soon be born. It is the event for which
you have been waiting and planning. If this is your first
pregnancy, you will be anxious and concerned that all
will go well and this is an understandable concern. The
onset of labour normally occurs in most women
between 38 and 42 weeks after the last period. It may
start on its own (spontaneous) or it may be started by
medical intervention (induced).

Spontaneous labour

There are clinical signs that herald the onset of labour
(see box on page 110). These may occur individually or
in combination and in any order.

   The first sign is usually the appearance of a 'show'.
This is a plug of jelly-like material or mucus and is
passed vaginally, sometimes with some blood. This
mucus is produced by the glands of the cervix and is
thought to act as a barrier to ascending infection (see
figure).

   A tear or rupture in your membranes may occur
(spontaneous rupture of the membranes or SRM).
When this happens there is a gush of amniotic fluid

The onset of labour

There are three main clinical signs that signal the start of labour:

1. Shedding of cervical plug – 'show'
2. Spontaneous rupture of the membranes – 'waters' break
3. Regular contractions start

The 'show'
During pregnancy the cervix is 'plugged' by a jelly-like material (a mucus plug), which is thought to help prevent infections. The first sign that labour is due to start is the appearance of a 'show' – the passing of this mucus plug.

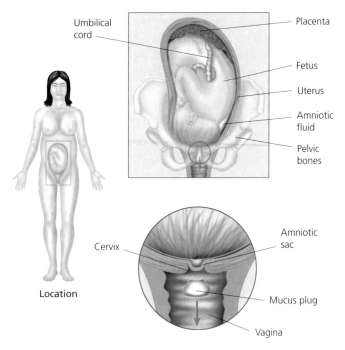

Location

Umbilical cord

Placenta

Fetus

Uterus

Amniotic fluid

Pelvic bones

Cervix

Amniotic sac

Mucus plug

Vagina

that may be a small or large amount. If there has only been a small leakage, it may be difficult to know if this is urine or amniotic fluid. The fluid tends to go on leaking, however, and you may soak several pads. If there is doubt, your doctor or midwife may do an internal examination using a speculum to see if amniotic fluid is passing through your cervix. Sometimes SRM occurs before your contractions start. If they do not then start within 24 hours, they are usually stimulated with medical preparations.

Contractions of the muscle of the uterus may start of their own accord before the appearance of show or SRM. They tend to be mild initially, occurring once or twice every 10 minutes and lasting for 20 to 40 seconds. Once labour is established, they will last for 40 to 60 seconds and occur three to five times every 10 minutes. Your doctor or midwife will give you a vaginal examination to assess your cervix. If the cervix is shortening in length (effacing) and dilating (widening), labour has begun.

Induction of labour

Labour is induced in 20 to 30 per cent of pregnancies. There are several reasons for this (see box on page 112). The most common reason is that the pregnancy has continued beyond 41 weeks. After this time, the risk of stillbirth (delivery of a dead fetus after week 24 of pregnancy) increases very slightly and it is considered safer to deliver the baby. The decision to induce a labour is normally taken after a full discussion of the reasons with the patient.

Methods of inducing labour

There are different methods of induction. Most commonly, if the cervix is found to be unfavourable (no sign of dilation after an internal examination), prostaglandins in the form of a tablet or gel are inserted into the upper vagina around the cervix. This hormone causes the uterus to contract and softens the cervix, making it more favourable. This process which takes several hours is referred to as ripening. Sometimes the onset of labour is triggered but, if this does not happen, then artificial rupture of the membranes (ARM or amniotomy) is undertaken.

ARM involves fingertip examination of your vagina (digital vaginal examination) and the passing of a small instrument called an amnihook (see figure on page 114), the size of a knitting needle, to hook and perforate your membranes. The procedure is painless in itself and all you will feel is the examining finger. It is much easier for you and the operator if you can relax your muscles to facilitate the examination. Following

Reasons for induction of labour

Labour may be induced for several reasons, for example:

- Post dates (overdue)
- Hypertension (high blood pressure)
- Diabetes
- Suspected small baby (intrauterine growth restricted or IUGR)
- Antepartum haemorrhage
- Maternal request

ARM, the amniotic fluid runs out of your vagina as in SRM and this may trigger your contractions.

If your contractions do not start or are weak, you will be given a hormone called Syntocinon to stimulate them (see page 115). It is given in solution through a drip placed in one of your arm veins. A low dose is given and increased every 15 minutes until your contractions are established.

Inducing labour: cervical ripening

The most common method to induce labour is to place a prostaglandin suppository into the upper vagina. Over a period of several hours, this hormone causes the cervix to relax and soften ('ripen'), making the cervix more likely to dilate.

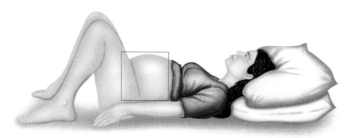

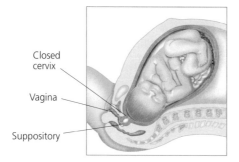

Closed cervix

Vagina

Suppository

Inducing labour: rupturing the membranes

If a suppository does not start labour, artificial rupturing of the membranes (ARM) is undertaken. The midwife or doctor examines the vagina with a fingertip. Then a small hook (amnihook) is passed up the vagina to perforate the amniotic sac and therefore trigger contractions.

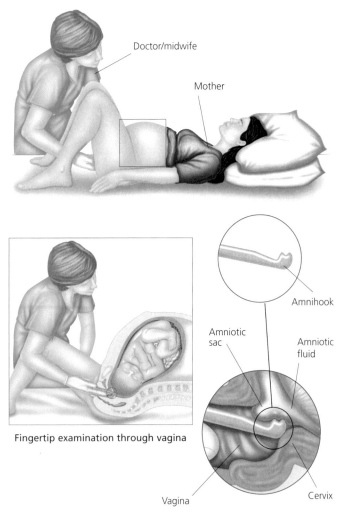

Doctor/midwife

Mother

Amnihook

Amniotic sac

Amniotic fluid

Fingertip examination through vagina

Vagina

Cervix

Inducing labour: hormonal stimulation

If your contractions do not start, yet the cervix is open and the membranes have ruptured, you will be given an intravenous dose of a hormone called Syntocinon. This should encourage the uterus to contract.

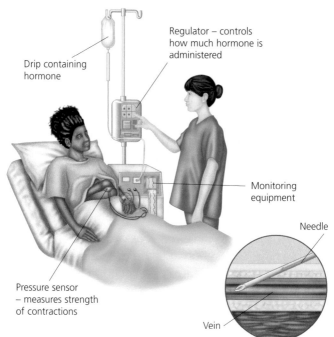

Drip containing hormone

Regulator – controls how much hormone is administered

Monitoring equipment

Pressure sensor – measures strength of contractions

Needle

Vein

The progress of labour

The length of labour tends to be longest in a first pregnancy. In the next one, the process has become more efficient. A first labour may last 12 to 24 hours but, in subsequent pregnancies, labour is usually shorter, perhaps lasting 6 to 12 hours. These are average figures. In present-day maternity care it is unusual for the active (see below) phase of labour to be much longer than 12 hours. There are three recognised stages of labour (see box on page 116).

The first stage

This is the longest stage and ends when the cervix becomes fully dilated. It consists of a latent phase and an active phase. During the latent phase, the contractions are mild but regular, occurring once every 5 to 10 minutes. It can be difficult to be certain that labour has started because the muscle of the uterus contracts intermittently every day throughout pregnancy. Sometimes bouts of contractions occur that may be painful but do not result in the onset of labour. These are called Braxton Hicks contractions.

The only way to be certain that labour has started is for your midwife or doctor to perform a vaginal examination. At the start of labour, the cervix shortens from two to three centimetres in length to less than one centimetre. This is called 'effacement'. The cervix also begins to dilate (widen) and when it is fully effaced and two to three centimetres dilated, the active phase begins. During this phase, labour becomes fully established with three to five good strength uterine contractions every 10 minutes, each contraction lasting 40 to 60 seconds.

The three stages of labour

Labour involves three distinct stages:

First stage: from onset of regular contractions to full dilation of the cervix

Second stage: from full dilation of the cervix to delivery of the baby

Third stage: from delivery of the baby to delivery of the placenta

Cervical changes

During labour, certain changes take place in the cervix: effacement (shortening) and dilation (widening).

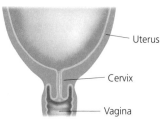

Uterus

Cervix

Vagina

Prelabour
Cervix is closed and long

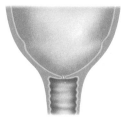

Effacement
Cervix shortens from 2 to 3 cm in length to less than 1 cm

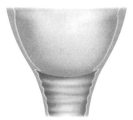

Dilation
Cervix dilates (widens)

Location

117

First stage of labour

The first stage of labour lasts from the onset of regular contractions to full dilation of the cervix. A vaginal examination is made periodically to assess the cervical dilation and position of the baby's head.

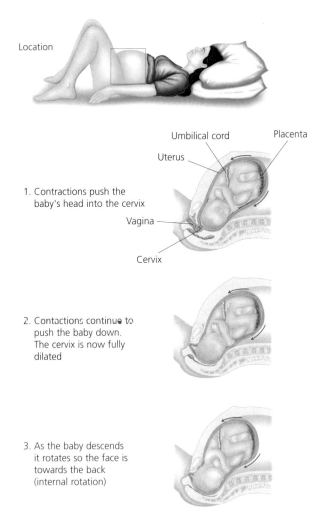

Location

Umbilical cord

Placenta

Uterus

1. Contractions push the baby's head into the cervix

Vagina

Cervix

2. Contractions continue to push the baby down. The cervix is now fully dilated

3. As the baby descends it rotates so the face is towards the back (internal rotation)

The progress of labour

The progress of labour is measured by assessing the strength and frequency of the uterine contractions, how far the fetal head has descended and how wide the cervix has dilated. A vaginal examination, usually every four hours, is used to assess the cervical dilation and the level of the head as it passes through the pelvis. The findings are charted on a partogram, which is a graph of parturition – the process of birth (see figure on page 120).

The partogram is a visual record of progress. On this chart the mother's temperature, urine output and analysis, pulse and blood pressure are recorded at regular intervals. The fetal heart rate is also documented along with the appearance of the amniotic fluid. Any medication and all intravenous fluids are noted. The partogram is supplemented with a carefully written record of the care given to the mother and fetus by the attending midwife and doctors.

The second stage

This does not normally last more than two hours and ends with delivery of your baby. During this time the head descends through your pelvis. You will experience a bearing down sensation – you feel that you need to push. Your midwife will guide, support and encourage you. This is an important time for you to give all the effort that you can to push your baby's head out. Normally your baby will be delivered within an hour of starting to push.

During this process the fetal head descends and passes through your pelvis. The head is naturally positioned transversely in keeping with the shape of

The partogram
The partogram is a complete visual record of measurements made during delivery.

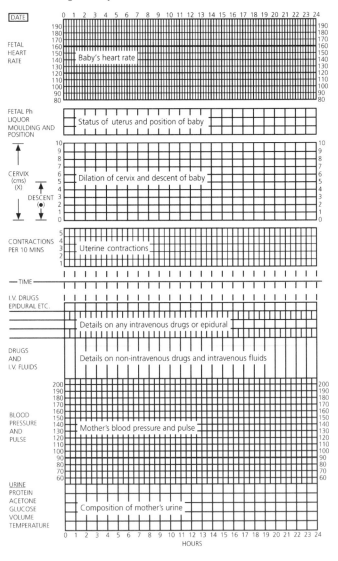

Second stage of labour

The second stage of labour lasts from full dilation of the cervix to delivery of the baby.

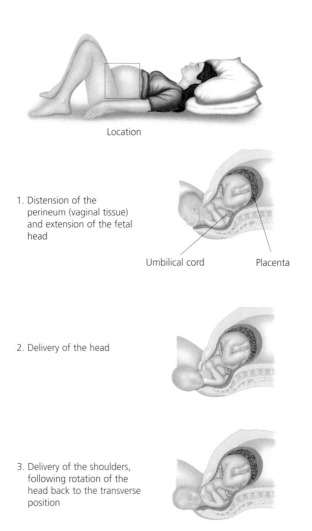

Location

1. Distension of the perineum (vaginal tissue) and extension of the fetal head

Umbilical cord   Placenta

2. Delivery of the head

3. Delivery of the shoulders, following rotation of the head back to the transverse position

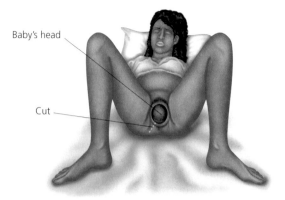

Baby's head

Cut

An episiotomy is a cut made in the skin to enlarge the vaginal opening. Having an episiotomy eases the passage of the baby and avoids tearing.

the pelvis. As it descends it rotates so that the face is towards the back. This is called internal rotation. The top or crown of the head then becomes visible to the attending midwife and begins to stretch the vaginal tissue as it delivers. This is called crowning.

The pain of the uterine contractions tends to be more than that of the delivery process. If your vagina is being stretched so much that crowning is delayed, an episiotomy may be needed (a cut made into the skin and muscle between the vagina and the anus to enlarge the birth opening). Local anaesthetic is injected into the area and a cut is made at the height of a contraction. Having an episiotomy allows easier passage of the baby and avoids tearing. The frequency of its use varies from unit to unit.

After the head has delivered (see figure on page 121), your midwife feels around your baby's neck to check that the umbilical cord is not around it. If the cord is there and is loose, it will be hooked over the head, but, if it is tight, it will be clamped and cut. The head naturally rotates back to the transverse position to allow the shoulders to pass through the pelvis. This is called external rotation. The anterior shoulder is then delivered with a further push and the rest of the body follows immediately.

The third stage

This does not normally last more than 30 minutes and ends with delivery of the placenta. There are two ways of doing this – active and passive management – with active management being the most commonly used.

Active management

In active management, as the shoulder is being delivered or immediately after the baby is born, an injection is given into your thigh muscle. This intramuscular injection contains two drugs, ergometrine and oxytocin, which

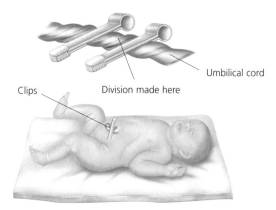

Umbilical cord

Clips   Division made here

Soon after your baby is born the umbilical cord is clamped by two clips and cut between them.

cause your uterus to contract, help the placenta to separate and reduce the blood loss. The two drugs are prepared in a vial and called Syntometrine. Soon after your baby is born, the umbilical cord is clamped by two metal clips and cut between them. For the cord that is still connected to the mother the midwife supports the uterus by placing her left hand on the abdomen (fundal pressure) and with her right hand pulls gently on the cord to encourage separation (see figure below). This is termed 'controlled cord traction' and, with this active management, the placenta and membranes should be delivered through the vagina within 30 minutes and blood loss is minimal – an average of 250 ml.

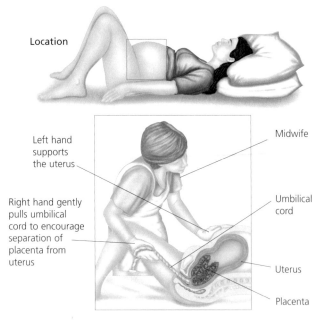

This illustration depicts 'active management' where the umbilical cord is gently pulled to encourage separation of the placenta from the uterus.

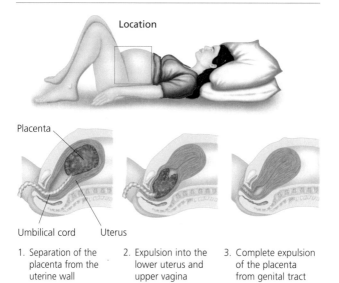

Location

Placenta

Umbilical cord   Uterus

1. Separation of the placenta from the uterine wall

2. Expulsion into the lower uterus and upper vagina

3. Complete expulsion of the placenta from genital tract

Passive management of the delivery of the placenta avoids the use of drugs, cord traction and fundal pressure. However, it is also associated with greater blood loss.

Passive management

Passive management avoids the use of drugs, cord traction and fundal pressure. Maternal effort and gravity work together to deliver the placenta, the cord being clamped and divided after it stops pulsating. This is associated with more blood loss and a greater need for transfusion. There is less risk of the nausea, vomiting and headache that Syntometrine may cause in some women. Some hospitals now use only Syntocinon to reduce this side effect.

Postpartum haemorrhage

In some women, severe haemorrhage (loss of blood) can occur after delivery. It is called postpartum haemorrhage (PPH) when the blood loss is more than

500 ml and can occur unexpectedly without any risk factors. This is one of the main reasons why obstetricians advise against home delivery. PPH can occur when the uterus relaxes after delivery of the baby, rather than continuing to contract and so putting pressure on the interior of the uterus. PPH may also occur if the birth passages are injured or the placenta not delivered (retained placenta). Again this prevents the natural control of bleeding by pressure.

In one to two per cent of deliveries, the placenta does not separate from the uterus because it is intricately interwoven within the wall of the uterus. The retained placenta has to be removed by an operation under spinal or general anaesthesia. During the procedure the obstetrician inserts a hand through the vagina inside the uterus and carefully separates the placenta from the wall of the uterus. This is termed 'manual removal of the placenta' and is usually effective.

Very rarely the placenta has implanted so deep into the muscle wall of the uterus (placenta accreta) that it has to be left behind. This is a serious condition with a significant risk of infection. Consequently careful medical follow-up and supervision are required.

Pain relief

The contractions of labour are painful. However, there are many things that can be done to reduce this pain (see box on page 128). The first is preparation for labour. Knowing in advance where you are going, what is going to happen and the options available for pain relief will help. Your midwife will give you great support, reassurance and advice during your labour. The presence of your partner or a close friend or relative can also give you support and reassurance.

Such things can relieve your anxiety and this is very important because there is a close link between anxiety and pain. If your anxiety levels are low you will find the experience less painful. Everyone has a different pain threshold and some patients find labour a terrible experience whereas others enjoy it. Much depends on your attitude beforehand.

Non-drug pain relief

There are several non-pharmacological methods that can be employed to relieve pain. Most of these are diversion therapy, aimed at taking your mind away from the pain. Listening to your favourite music, massage by your partner, walking or changing your position all help. More involved alternative methods are aromatherapy, acupuncture and hypnosis. These are unlikely to be available unless you make arrangements yourself. Hypnosis may be in the form of self-hypnosis where you go into a state of trance, using relaxation, visualisation and distraction. Posthypnotic suggestion can also be used where you have previously seen a hypnotist who programmes you for labour.

In early labour, the contractions are less strong and frequent, so less pain relief is required. As the contractions become stronger, a warm bath may help. Transcutaneous electrical nerve stimulation (TENS) is a method of pain relief in which small electrodes are placed on the skin of your back on either side of your spine. Electrical impulses are given which cause a buzzing or tingling sensation that alleviates the pain of the contractions. The intensity of the impulses can be changed.

Methods of pain relief

There are several ways to reduce labour pain, either using drugs or trying other self-help measures.

Non-drug
- Music
- Movement/support and position
- Warm bath
- Massage
- Aromatherapy
- Hypnosis
- Acupuncture
- TENS (transcutaneous electrical nerve stimulation)

Drugs
- Entonox
- Pethidine/morphine/diamorphine
- Epidural

Pain relief with drugs

The drug options fall into several categories: Entonox, intramuscular opiates, epidural anaesthetic and spinal anaesthetic.

Entonox

This is a mixture of nitrous oxide and oxygen given by facemask. It is often referred to as gas and air; it is very safe and takes the edge off the pain. It is also useful when the contractions are beginning to become painful or in late first stage and second stage when it is too late for other forms of pain relief.

Intramuscular opiates

Drugs such as pethidine and morphine should be

requested once the contractions are really painful. These are the most powerful pain-relieving drugs available. They may cause nausea and vomiting and an anti-nausea drug (anti-emetic) can be given to reduce this side effect. They are normally given at four-hourly intervals because overdosage will suppress your breathing and also have an effect on the baby's breathing at birth. Drugs can be given to the baby to reverse such sedative effects if delivery happens soon after you have been given an opiate.

Epidural anaesthetic

If none of these methods is effective, an epidural anaesthetic can be given. An anaesthetist injects a local anaesthetic into the epidural space that surrounds your spinal cord (see figure on page 130). This blocks the pain sensations coming from the uterus and vagina. It takes about 30 minutes to administer and about 30 minutes to be effective, so timing is important to relate to how long it is thought that you will have to go before delivery.

The procedure is usually straightforward and gives great pain relief. Sometimes the insertion can be difficult because the epidural space, which is accessed between two of the bones in your lower back (the lumbar vertebrae), cannot be easily found for the injection. This can result in an incomplete block that gives some but not total pain relief. Occasionally, a dural tap can occur when the needle passes into the spinal canal and some of the fluid around the spine leaks into the epidural space. This can cause severe headache. After delivery, if the headache is troublesome, the anaesthetist may inject a little of your blood into the epidural space to 'patch' or seal the small hole.

The use of epidural anaesthesia is associated with an increased use of assisted delivery techniques because

Epidural anaesthesia

Epidural anaesthesia is a very effective form of pain relief for labour. It involves the injection of local anaesthetic agents into the lumbar epidural space (which surrounds the spinal cord).

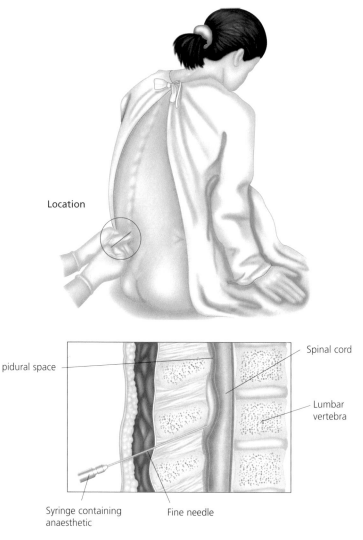

Location

pidural space

Spinal cord

Lumbar vertebra

Syringe containing anaesthetic

Fine needle

most of the labours are longer and more tiring for the patient. There are no proven short- or long-term problems associated with epidural anaesthesia.

Spinal anaesthetic
A spinal anaesthetic is the usual method of anaesthesia for caesarean section (see page 139). It entails a single injection through a very fine needle of local anaesthetic directly into the spinal canal. Its effect is more immediate and it does not last as long as an epidural.

Fetal monitoring and fetal distress
The condition of the fetus is checked or monitored during labour by various methods to assess that enough oxygen is being received. When this is not the case, the lack of oxygen (hypoxia) will cause fetal distress. During the contractions of labour, the blood flow and oxygen supply from the mother to the placenta are reduced and in some labours this may cause hypoxia in the fetus. It is important to detect hypoxia because, if it lasts for a long time, it may cause injury to the organs of the fetus.

Checking the amniotic fluid
The first method employed is to assess the colour of the amniotic fluid that is being passed. This is normally clear but, if the fetus becomes distressed, it will be green. This is called meconium staining of the amniotic fluid and is the result of the fetus passing a bowel motion into the fluid. The bowel motion is called meconium and it has a green slimy consistency. Meconium staining is not always a sign of fetal distress and is also seen in labour when there has been none. It is more common in pregnancies that have gone beyond 40 weeks.

Fetal heart rate monitoring

During labour, the condition of the baby is checked. If a heart rate abnormality is suspected or there is a risk that fetal distress will occur, a continuous recording of the fetal heart rate is taken. The measurements can be taken externally through the mother's abdomen or by attaching a clip to the baby's head (more accurate).

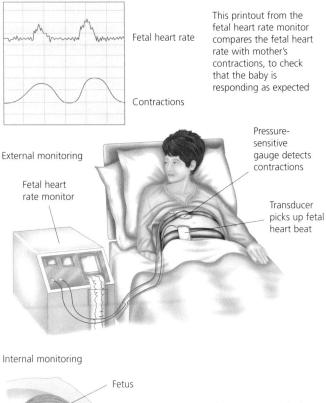

Fetal heart rate

Contractions

This printout from the fetal heart rate monitor compares the fetal heart rate with mother's contractions, to check that the baby is responding as expected

External monitoring

Fetal heart rate monitor

Pressure-sensitive gauge detects contractions

Transducer picks up fetal heart beat

Internal monitoring

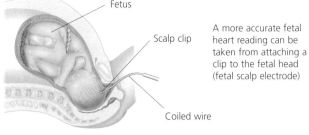

Fetus

Scalp clip

A more accurate fetal heart reading can be taken from attaching a clip to the fetal head (fetal scalp electrode)

Coiled wire

Checking the fetal heart rate

The second method is to listen to the fetal heart rate at regular intervals between contractions. This used to be performed with a stethoscope but now the attending midwife more commonly uses an electronic hand-held monitor to pick up the sound of the heart beat. It is the rate of the fetal heart that is important and this is normally between 110 and 160 beats per minute.

Continuous monitoring

When there is any suspicion of a heart rate abnormality or if there are risk factors in labour that may make fetal distress more likely, a continuous record of the heart rate is preferred. This is done either externally with a small plastic disc (transducer) strapped to the mother's abdomen or internally by attaching a short coiled wire (a fetal scalp electrode) to the fetal head. A read-out of the heart rate is printed on a trace, which also records the contractions. This tracing is called a cardiotocograph or CTG.

The heart rate is recorded continuously and in particular the response to contractions. The heart rate may fall with a contraction (deceleration) and the onset of the decelerations may be early, variable or late in relation to the onset of the contraction. This observation is important because late decelerations are associated with fetal hypoxia. Variable decelerations are the result of cord compression and may cause hypoxia. Early decelerations are caused by head compression, commonly seen in second stage, and are not associated with hypoxia.

Further tests

When there is a suspicious fetal heart rate pattern, further methods are required to assess whether the fetus is hypoxic. This is done by taking a small pinprick of blood from the top of the head of the fetus which is presenting in the vagina. This is called fetal blood sampling and the acidity is measured in this blood to assess whether the fetus is getting enough oxygen. If the fetal heart rate pattern is very bad, this final test may not be done and the baby will be delivered immediately. This will be by caesarean section or assisted vaginally if the cervix is fully dilated.

Abnormal labour and assisted delivery

Sometimes a labour fails to progress. This is a result of problems with the 'powers', 'passenger' or 'passages' (see box opposite). The powers are the uterine contractions and, during the second stage, the maternal effort required to push the baby out through the birth canal. Either or both of these may be too weak to be effective.

The passenger is the fetus that may be too large or presenting abnormally, such as bottom first (breech). If the breech presentation had been discovered before labour, an attempt to turn the fetus to head first would normally be discussed with you. This is called external cephalic version (ECV) and is normally undertaken at about 37 weeks. The obstetrician examines the abdomen to locate the bottom and the head of the fetus. Manual pressure is then applied, clockwise or anti-clockwise, to rotate the fetus (version) to the cephalic presentation. It has a 30 per cent success rate in a first pregnancy and 60 per cent in women who have had previous deliveries. If the ECV is successful, it reduces the need for caesarean section which is the preferred method of delivery for a fetus presenting by breech.

Sometimes the head may be in the wrong position and present a larger diameter that will have difficulty passing through the pelvis. The passages are the pelvis and soft tissues. The bony pelvis may be too small or there may be a large ovarian cyst that can obstruct the birth canal.

The most common problem is that the uterine contractions are too weak. An intravenous preparation can be given that will increase the strength of the contractions. This is called Syntocinon and it is given in low doses that are increased to a maximum level. It has to be given carefully at fixed infusion rates because too much can result in contractions that are too strong.

If progress remains insufficient despite Syntocinon, assistance will be required. If the second stage has not been reached, the baby will be delivered by caesarean section. If the second stage has been reached, delivery can be assisted by a vacuum (Ventouse) or forceps. In competent hands these techniques do not harm the baby. Maternal effort is still required.

Sometimes the head may not be low enough in the birth canal for assisted vaginal delivery to be safe

Abnormal labour

Labour may fail to progress for several reasons:

- **Powers:** contractions; maternal effort insufficient to push baby out
- **Passenger:** large baby; abnormal presentation – for example, bottom first; fetal distress
- **Passages:** pelvis too small; soft tissue obstruction

enough and the operator has to opt for a caesarean section.

Vaginal delivery is considered safer than either planned (elective) or emergency caesarean section. A caesarean section is an abdominal operation performed under an anaesthetic. It carries an increased risk of haemorrhage, blood transfusion, wound infection and blood clot formation (thrombosis) in the leg veins.

Apart from failure of labour to progress, the second most common reason for an emergency caesarean section is fetal distress – when abnormalities are detected in the fetal heart rate pattern.

Methods of assisted delivery
Vacuum extraction

A small metal or soft plastic cup is used to assist delivery in the second stage of labour. Pain relief with local anaesthetic is always used to freeze the skin around the vagina. A further injection of local anaesthetic may be given inside the vagina to anaesthetise the two nerves that are responsible for sensation around the vagina and perineal area. These are called the pudendal nerves and the method of anaesthesia is called a pudendal nerve block. Often an epidural has been given earlier in labour and this may be 'topped up' with more local anaesthetic. Occasionally a spinal anaesthetic is given.

The operator empties the bladder with a catheter, undertakes a vaginal examination to confirm that the cervix is fully dilated, determines the position of the head, and checks that it is far enough down in the vagina to ensure that safe delivery can be attempted. The cup is then applied to the fetal head. There is a thin rubber tube leading from the cup to a pump which creates a vacuum between the cup and the fetal head. There is a pressure gauge which informs the operator when enough vacuum has been created. The operator pulls on the rubber tubing attached to the cup to exert traction on the head and assist delivery. The traction is undertaken only during a contraction when the maternal effort of pushing reduces the traction force required. It may take up to five or six contractions before the baby is delivered.

At delivery, the baby's head will have an elongated shape where the vacuum cup has been applied and there

Vacuum (Ventouse) delivery

A suction cup (Ventouse) is applied to the baby's head. Air is extracted from the suction cup to create a vacuum and stick the cup to the head. The cup is then pulled to assist the delivery of the baby.

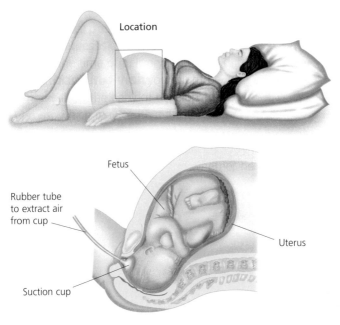

Location

Fetus

Rubber tube
to extract air
from cup

Uterus

Suction cup

will be bruising in the underlying tissues. This disappears within a day or so and rarely causes any problems.

An episiotomy is usually undertaken to aid the delivery (see page 122).

Forceps delivery

As with vacuum delivery, the bladder is emptied, pain relief given and the vagina examined. It is important that the operator determines the position of the fetal head because the forceps have to be placed accurately on either side. Most forceps deliveries are undertaken when the head is in the correct position, with the back of the fetal head (the occiput) towards the front of the mother. This position is called occipitoanterior.

Forceps delivery

Metal forceps are inserted into the vagina and placed on either side of the baby's head. The doctor/midwife pulls with the forceps as the mother pushes the baby out.

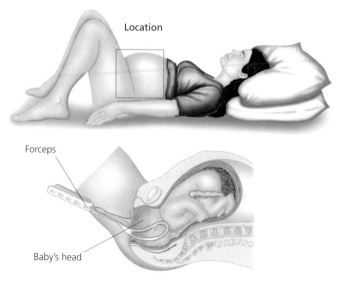

Location

Forceps

Baby's head

Between contractions the forceps blades are applied. They are then locked together. With the next contraction, the mother is asked to push and the operator pulls on the forceps to deliver the head. The head is normally delivered over one or two contractions. An episiotomy is always made to avoid any tears of the vagina.

If the head is not in the correct position (malpositioned), a rotational forceps delivery is required. A different type of forceps is used for this procedure, which requires more skill on the part of the operator. Many doctors now prefer using the vacuum to forceps because the risk of maternal injury is less.

Occasionally, the head will fail to descend despite the assisted effort and a caesarean section is then required to deliver the baby.

Caesarean section

Caesarean (C) section is undertaken either as a planned (elective) procedure or as an emergency. Twenty to thirty per cent of babies are delivered by C section and most doctors and midwives consider this too high. There are complex reasons for the increase in this rate over the last 10 years which are a combination of patients' wishes and doctors' concerns about the well-being of the fetus and mother. It is unusual for a patient in a first pregnancy to have an elective C section unless the baby is presenting by breech or there is another significant complication. Most women who have a C section in their first pregnancy have this performed as an emergency because of fetal distress or failure to progress satisfactorily in labour.

An elective C section is normally planned to be undertaken at 39 weeks. If it is done before this time there is a slightly increased risk that the baby may have breathing difficulties, requiring admission to the neonatal unit for observation. The operation is usually performed under spinal anaesthetic. This means that the woman and her partner can be awake to see the delivery of the baby. Admission is usually the day before planned surgery. This is also an opportunity to meet the anaesthetist, obstetrician, midwives and theatre staff. Consent for the operation must be obtained. A blood sample will be taken for grouping to cross-match, and an antacid given before the operation to reduce the acidity in the stomach in case

Breech birth

If the baby is lying with its bottom closest to the cervix, this is said to be a 'breech birth' and is a common reason for a caesarean section.

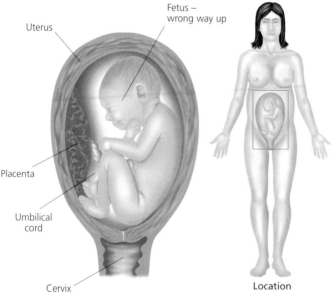

Uterus

Fetus – wrong way up

Placenta

Umbilical cord

Cervix

Location

the patient is sick. Some of the pubic hair will be shaved so that the incision on the skin is made along or below the 'bikini line'. Admission can be arranged for the day of the operation but it is important that no food or fluids are taken for at least six hours before the operation.

When in theatre, a drip is placed in one of the arm veins and the blood pressure and pulse are recorded

Caesarean section

In a caesarean section, the baby is delivered through an incision in the mother's abdominal wall rather than through the vagina.

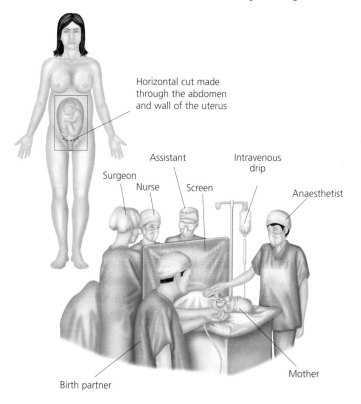

Horizontal cut made through the abdomen and wall of the uterus

Assistant

Intravenous drip

Surgeon

Nurse

Screen

Anaesthetist

Mother

Birth partner

with monitors. This is necessary before the spinal anaesthetic is put in. A catheter is then placed in the bladder and inflatable rubber leggings are placed around the legs to reduce the risk of blood clot forming in the leg veins (thrombosis). The skin is cleansed and sterile covers applied.

As the patient is lying flat the operation is not seen by her or her seated partner. However, when the baby is delivered the obstetrician holds it up so that it is immediately visible. The baby is then normally handed to the midwife or paediatrician for initial inspection. It only takes about 5 to 10 minutes to deliver the baby and after that another 30 minutes or so to close the wounds on the uterus, the muscle and skin of the abdomen. During the operation, antibiotics are given to reduce the risk of infection, and afterwards heparin may be given to thin the blood and reduce the risk of thrombosis.

After the operation, two to three hours are spent in a recovery area where the blood pressure, pulse and wound site are checked and any heavy vaginal bleeding recorded. Pain relief is usually given through the drip and controlled by the patient (patient-controlled analgesia or PCA). During this time the baby is examined and weighed. The wound takes about a week to heal and obviously the patient feels discomfort for a week or two. Feeling on the skin around the wound never returns to normal. Unfortunately, driving is not advisable for six weeks after a C section. You should check with your car insurance if you wish to drive before this time.

An emergency C section does not always have to be performed in haste and in most instances there is time to prepare the patient and her partner psychologically for the event. This preparation involves support for the couple to reduce the possible disappointment at not having achieved a vaginal delivery or the anxiety for the well-being of the unborn child and mother. In most instances the operation is performed with the mother awake and her partner in attendance. If an epidural anaesthetic is already in place it will require 'topping up' to increase the anaesthetised area to above the umbilicus. Alternatively a spinal or, more rarely, a general anaesthetic may be given.

KEY POINTS

■ The onset of labour may be spontaneous or induced

■ Labour has three stages: in the first, the progress of labour is assessed by cervical dilation and descent of the head; in the second contractions and maternal effort deliver the baby; and in the third the placenta is delivered

■ Spontaneous vertex (head first with the crown of the head leading the way) is the normal mode of delivery

■ Delivery may be assisted by vacuum, forceps or caesarean section

■ The placenta usually follows within 30 minutes of delivery and the average blood loss is 250 ml

■ Preparation for labour is important to reduce anxiety and the need for pain relief

Postnatal problems

The postnatal period
The first six weeks after delivery is referred to as the postnatal period or puerperium. This is the time when your body gradually returns to its pre-pregnant state and the hormonal influences of pregnancy are withdrawn. During this time, it is normal to have some mild problems that are not life threatening. Occasionally more serious problems can develop that require medical supervision.

After pains
Your uterus continues to contract after delivery as it returns to its normal state. In the first few days you may experience afterbirth pains that are the result of these contractions. They are particularly noticeable when you begin to breast-feed, which stimulates the release of hormones from the pituitary gland. If they are very painful paracetamol tablets will help.

Perineal pain
Your vagina and underlying tissues become more elastic and vascular in late pregnancy, in preparation for the delivery of your baby. The area between your vagina and back passage is called the perineum.

During delivery the perineal tissues are stretched and may tear. Sometimes a cut, called an episiotomy, is necessary to reduce the risk of tearing and ease the delivery of the head. After local anaesthetic has been injected, the episiotomy is made with sharp scissors at the height of a contraction. The episiotomy will need a stitched repair, as will any significant tears. Stitching helps reduce blood loss and aids healing.

It is normal to experience discomfort and some pain in the perineal area even if you have no stitches. About one in ten patients still has perineal discomfort after four months. There are several remedies that you can try (see box below). There is little clinical evidence of proven benefit but as an individual you may find something that works for you.

A warm bath is a great comfort. This will probably have to wait until you go home because hospitals tend to have showers, which are better for infection control. The addition of salt, Savlon or lavender oil to the bath water may help, but has not been shown to be of benefit.

Managing perineal pain

Tearing or cutting of the perineal tissues (between the vagina and back passage) can cause discomfort. This can be eased by:

- Having a warm bath
- Applying ice packs
- Using local anaesthetic sprays and gels
- Applying gauze swab soaked in witch hazel
- Doing pelvic floor exercises
- Taking painkillers

Local applications to the perineum may help. These are short-lived but do give some relief. Ice packs are the most common recommendation and cause numbing. Carefully sitting for a short time on a bag of frozen peas can give great relief. Local anaesthetic sprays and gels (aqueous five per cent lignocaine/ lidocaine) may be used. Gauze swabs or pads soaked in witch hazel, applied to the perineal area, have been used but tap water has been shown to be equally good.

It can help to reduce the pressure on the sore area by sitting on a support cushion, wedge or pillow. A physiotherapist can help with suggestions – for example, pelvic floor exercises have been proved to reduce pain at three months after delivery. The more expensive treatments of ultrasound or pulsed electromagnetic energy have not been proved.

Oral painkillers (analgesics) can alleviate a painful perineum, particularly in the first week or two after delivery. Paracetamol is the best analgesic for this and the normal dose is free of unwanted side effects. Ibuprofen is a suitable alternative. A small dose of codeine may be added but it can cause constipation. Aspirin is less good because it increases bleeding time and is excreted in breast milk.

Haemorrhoids (piles) are itchy, painful dilated veins that protrude through the anus. They are caused by the increased pressure in the pelvis and are common in late pregnancy (see page 83). They disappear after pregnancy but this may be a painful process. The same remedies suggested for new piles can help and local anaesthetic creams or suppositories can also give relief.

Lochia, infection and haemorrhage

Lochia is the normal discharge of blood and mucus that is passed from the vagina after delivery. It comes from the lining of the uterus. It is heavy like a menstrual period for the first couple of days, becomes light and pink for a week, and finally pale yellow for another week or so.

If it has an offensive smell or appears to contain pus, you may have endometritis (inflammation or infection of the lining of the uterus) and need to take antibiotics. If fever develops, it is a serious condition called puerperal fever. It used to be a common cause of death after delivery but, fortunately, with the use of antibiotics, this is now rare.

If the bleeding becomes very heavy, you will need medical attention. If excessive bleeding occurs within 24 hours of delivery this is known as primary postpartum haemorrhage and may be the result of relaxation of the uterine muscle, an unstitched tear within the vagina or retained placental tissue. Bleeding beyond this time is called secondary postpartum haemorrhage and may be caused by retained placental tissue or endometritis.

Phlebitis and deep vein thrombosis

Varicose veins are very common in pregnancy as a result of pooling of blood in the leg veins, which results from the pressure effects of the increased weight of the pregnancy and the fetus within the pelvis. The veins may become large and tortuous and may be painful if you stand for a long time (see page 85).

After delivery the pressure is suddenly reduced and the veins become less congested. This sometimes sets off an inflammatory response in the vessel wall and they appear inflamed with the red outline of the vein seen on the surface of the leg. This is called phlebitis. Occasionally, a blood clot may form in the surface vein causing thrombophlebitis. These normally settle without any treatment and, as long as the problem is in the surface veins, there is no health risk.

A painful, swollen leg may be a sign that a blood clot has formed in the deep veins in the leg or pelvis (deep vein thrombosis or DVT). This is a serious problem because the clot may become dislodged. It may be swept along with the venous blood returning to your heart and then to your lungs – a condition called a pulmonary embolism. This causes severe chest pain and

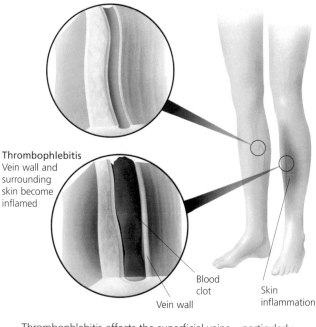

Thrombophlebitis
Vein wall and surrounding skin become inflamed

Blood clot

Skin inflammation

Vein wall

Thrombophlebitis affects the superficial veins – particularly varicose veins.

breathlessness and is a life-threatening condition which needs urgent medical help. If a DVT is suspected, your leg veins will be investigated with Doppler ultrasound. Treatment will be given to reduce the risk of further blood clots forming or being swept into the lungs.

The baby blues and postnatal depression

About half of all women who give birth experience 'baby blues'. This occurs in the first week after birth – usually the second or third day when all your friends and relatives are happy for you and the baby, but you do not feel the same. The feeling is a brief but intense one of misery and tearfulness. It is more common in first pregnancies.

Postnatal depression is less common, affecting 10 to 15 women in every 1,000 who give birth. It may be mild, or more severe, requiring antidepressant medication. Symptoms include difficulty concentrating (simple tasks take enormous effort), exhaustion on wakening, feeling a failure, numbness, laughing less and tearfulness. Patients are often reluctant to seek help because they feel guilty and a failure, and that people will regard them as unfit to raise a child.

However, it is important to seek early help because the response to treatment is good and will benefit your relationships with baby and partner. Certain risk factors for postnatal depression are recognised and health workers are becoming more vigilant of the problem. Testing for depression may be offered at six weeks and/or three months after delivery. This is becoming a routine in which you answer a set of questions. The Edinburgh Postnatal Depression Scale is widely used for this purpose (see box on pages 152–3). A cut-off score greater than 9 suggests 'possible depression' and more than 12 suggests 'probable depression'.

About 1 to 2 women per 1,000 suffer from puerperal psychosis after birth – a severe illness requiring psychiatric treatment. It is characterised by mood disorder, loss of contact with reality and abnormal behaviour with hallucinations. Risk factors include a past history of mental illness requiring hospital admission, previous puerperal psychosis and a family history of psychotic illness. Specialist review should be given to patients at risk.

Your baby
Condition at birth

It is normal practice for you to see your baby immediately at birth. Normally, the baby cries soon after delivery. The baby's skin will be wet with amniotic fluid and some of your blood. There will also be a coating of 'vernix' that resembles cream cheese. Its function was to protect the baby's skin when it was bathed in amniotic fluid. After the cord is clamped and divided, the baby is gently dried with a towel. This is to reduce heat loss from being wet. You can then hold your baby allowing skin-to-skin contact while covered in a warm blanket.

Sometimes a baby does not cry immediately and may appear blue. The baby's condition is 'scored' at around one and five minutes after birth. This scoring is named after the paediatrician, Virginia Apgar, who described it (see page 154). If your baby has poor Apgar scores, then he or she may need resuscitation. This takes the form of clearing the airways of mucus with suction, giving oxygen by facemask and, in rare cases, passing a tube to ventilate the lungs. If you have had a narcotic analgesic, such as pethidine, for pain relief, this can sometimes have a sedative effect on the

Edinburgh postnatal depression scale

Testing for depression is becoming routine after delivery. You may be asked a set of questions, such as the following. For this test a score greater than 9 suggests 'possible depression', and more than 12 'probable depression'.

1 I have been able to laugh and see the funny side of things:

As much as I always could	0
Not quite so much now	1
Definitely not so much now	2
Not at all	3

2 I have looked forward with enjoyment to things:

As much as I ever did	0
Rather less than I used to	1
Definitely less than I used to	2
Hardly at all	3

3 I have blamed myself unnecessarily when things went wrong:

Yes, most of the time	3
Yes, some of the time	2
Not very often	1
No, never	0

4 I have felt worried and anxious for no very good reason:

No, not at all	0
Hardly ever	1
Yes, sometimes	2
Yes, very often	3

5 I have felt scared or panicky for no very good reason:

Yes, quite a lot	3
Yes, sometimes	2
No, not much	1
No, not at all	0

Edinburgh postnatal depression scale (contd)

6 Things have been getting on top of me:
Yes, most of the time I haven't been able to
   cope at all   3
Yes, sometimes I haven't been coping as
   well as usual   2
No, most of the time I have coped quite well   1
No, I have been coping as well as ever   0

**7 I have been so unhappy that I have
had difficulty sleeping:**
Yes, most of the time   3
Yes, some of the time   2
Not very often   1
No, not at all   0

8 I have felt sad or miserable:
Yes, most of the time   3
Yes, some of the time   2
Not very often   1
No, not at all   0

**9 I have been so unhappy that I have
been crying:**
Yes, most of the time   3
Yes, quite often   2
Only occasionally   1
No, never   0

**10 The thought of harming myself has
occurred to me:**
Yes, quite often   3
Sometimes   2
Hardly ever   1
Never   0

The Apgar scores

A newborn baby's condition is 'scored' around one minute and then again five minutes after birth.

Criteria	For example	
	1 minute	5 minutes
Skin colour (0 = pale and blue, 1 = blue extremities, 2 = pink)	1	2
Muscle tone (0 = limp, 1 = moves limbs, 2 = good)	1	2
Respiratory effort (0 = none, 1 = gasps, 2 = good)	2	2
Heart rate (0 = none, 1 < 100, 2 > 100)	1	2
Response to stimulus (0 = none, 1 = slight, 2 = good	1	2
Total score out of 10 =	6	10

baby. This sedative action can be reversed by giving the baby a drug called naloxone.

Sometimes the amniotic fluid may have been stained with meconium, the bowel content of the fetus before delivery. This can be quite toxic to the newborn baby if inhaled so, if meconium-stained amniotic fluid is present at delivery, the paediatrician or midwife will ensure that the airways are clear of any of this fluid. This is usually done using suction through a thin plastic tube.

Vitamin K

It is standard practice to give an injection of vitamin K to the baby very soon after birth to reduce the risk of haemorrhagic disease of the newborn. This is a serious condition that can present as bleeding under the skin, from the cord or bowels or into the brain. Its incidence has been reduced by the use of vitamin K given as an intramuscular injection. There has been no proved adverse effect for this practice and it has been undertaken routinely for almost 40 years.

Feeding

There is clear scientific evidence that breast-feeding is better than bottle feeding. Breast milk contains the ideal fluid and nutrient content for your baby during the first four to six months of life. It also contains antibodies that give protection against many infections, especially gastroenteritis. Mothers who breast-feed also have a reduced risk of ovarian and premenopausal breast cancer.

Although breast-feeding is a natural thing to do, both mother and baby have to learn how to do it. Some practical and emotional support are necessary to make this a satisfying and enjoyable experience for both mother and baby. An understanding of the physiology of lactation is helpful (see figure on page 156).

Immediately after delivery, further hormonal changes occur. Prolactin from the pituitary gland of the mother's brain influences the breast glandular tissue to produce milk. Whenever a baby feeds further prolactin is released into the bloodstream stimulating the milk-producing cells so that they produce more milk. This milk gathers in the small ducts and sinuses. When the baby's mouth attaches to the nipple, a reflex ejection of milk occurs. This is brought about by the release of oxytocin from the pituitary, which causes the ducts in the breast to contract and eject the milk to the larger channels under the nipple. The suction applied by the

Hormonal control of breast-feeding

Two hormones are released when your baby feeds. Prolactin stimulates the breast glandular tissue to produce milk. Oxytocin causes the ducts in the breast to contract and eject milk.

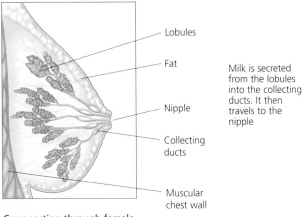

Lobules

Fat

Nipple

Collecting ducts

Muscular chest wall

Milk is secreted from the lobules into the collecting ducts. It then travels to the nipple

Cross-section through female breast

baby then draws the milk out of the breast. The more the baby feeds the more milk is produced.

Babies have different needs after birth and will not all be hungry at the same time. Trying to breast-feed your baby within the first two hours of birth is ideal but it is best not to be strict about when and when not to breast-feed. Privacy for the first feed helps so that you and your baby are relaxed and comfortable. Skilled professional help should be available from the team who delivered your baby. Try not to give additional fluids or artificial feeds to your baby and drink fluids whenever you want.

The most crucial element to successful breast-feeding is correct positioning. Your baby should be turned towards your breast with the nostrils or top lip opposite your nipple (see figure below). When attachment at the breast takes place, the bottom lip should be further away from your nipple than the top lip. The chin should come into contact with your breast first. In this way, your baby's mouth is around and mostly under your nipple area at the moment the mouth gapes. Such correct positioning ensures pain-free and effective feeding, and is important to avoid cracked nipples. There is no medical evidence to show that you need to toughen up or break in your nipples for feeding.

For the first day or so you should not restrict the frequency of feeds – they may be at intervals of one to eight hours. Nor should you restrict the duration of

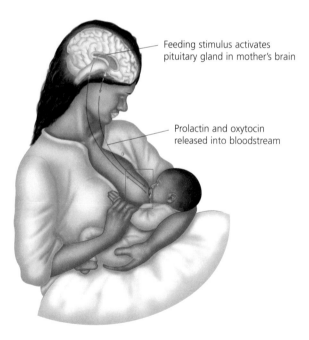

Feeding stimulus activates pituitary gland in mother's brain

Prolactin and oxytocin released into bloodstream

feeding. Such a flexible approach is important to reduce the risk of problems such as nipple trauma, engorgement or inflammation of the breasts (mastitis), and insufficient milk.

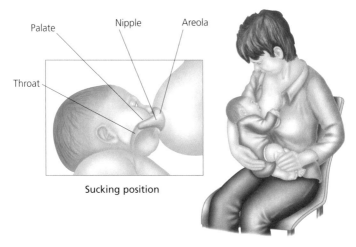

Palate   Nipple   Areola

Throat

Sucking position

This is the most crucial element to successful – and pain-free – breast-feeding. The entire nipple needs to be taken into the baby's mouth, for effective breast-feeding.

KEY POINTS

- The postnatal period or puerperium lasts for six weeks after delivery

- 'After pains', perineal pain, breast tenderness and the 'baby blues' are common problems

- Haemorrhage, infection and deep vein thrombosis are rare but serious complications

- Early detection of postnatal depression is important

- Your baby's condition at birth is always assessed with Apgar scores at one and five minutes

- Breast-feeding is best for your baby

Pregnancy loss

Miscarriage

The loss of a wanted pregnancy through miscarriage is a very distressing experience, regardless of gestation. Some women recover quickly but others may experience significant grief. Coping with the grief may be difficult and feelings of sadness, anger, loneliness and depression are not unusual. It will help if you can communicate and share your grief and feelings with your partner. It may also help to share your feelings with close friends or relatives. In addition, the Miscarriage Association can be contacted (see page 176) and will give support and advice to anyone who is in need.

Risk factors for miscarriage

Miscarriage is more common than is generally appreciated and complicates approximately one in five pregnancies. Miscarriage is the loss of a pregnancy before viability. It most commonly occurs in the first three months of pregnancy but can occur up to 24 weeks, which is the gestational age of viability. Risk factors include age over 35 years, autoimmune disorders, poorly controlled diabetes and a history of several previous miscarriages.

About 50 per cent of miscarriages are the result of an abnormality in the chromosome make-up of the embryo. Other causes include immunological incompatibility between mother and fetus, infection, hormonal disorder or structural abnormality in the pelvic organs.

In most instances, investigation into the cause of the miscarriage is not undertaken unless there is recurrent miscarriage, which is usually defined as three or more miscarriages. Recurrent miscarriage may be the result of a chromosomal abnormality (unbalanced translocation) in one of the parents (see page 13) or autoantibodies in the mother. In most instances of recurrent miscarriage, no known cause is found.

Clinical signs of miscarriage

The clinical features of miscarriage vary. Typically, a pregnant woman may experience vaginal bleeding. At this stage it is called a threatened miscarriage. If uterine cramps also occur, it may be that the cervix is beginning to dilate. If this is the case, the miscarriage is inevitable.

Tissue in the form of products of conception may be passed. If all the products are passed, the miscarriage is termed complete. If not all of the products are passed, the miscarriage is termed incomplete and treatment will be given to complete the emptying of the uterus.

However, not all non-viable pregnancies miscarry immediately and, nowadays, most are diagnosed by ultrasound. It may be discovered during a routine early pregnancy scan or there may be a history of vaginal brown discharge, fresh bleeding or loss of pregnancy symptoms. If the pregnancy is non-viable, there will be no fetal heart pulsation seen during the ultrasound investigation. Occasionally, the pregnancy sac is seen but there is no identifiable embryo. This is termed an 'anembryonic pregnancy' or 'blighted ovum'.

Diagnosing non-viable pregnancy

There are strict criteria used to diagnose fetal or embryonic death and an anembryonic pregnancy. This is to ensure that there is no risk of confusion with an early viable pregnancy. The diagnoses are made as follows.

Anembryonic pregnancy

This is when the pregnancy sac measures more than 20 mm and there is no fetal pole (thickening of the area of the blastocyst that will go on to form the embryo) within the sac.

Fetal or embryonic death

This is when the crown–rump length is greater than 6 mm and there is no visible heartbeat.

Management of a miscarriage

After the ultrasound diagnosis of a non-viable pregnancy, the management options must be discussed. The pregnancy may be managed conservatively, allowing a natural miscarriage to occur. In some cases this may take several days and many patients opt to have treatment to evacuate the uterine contents. This may be done either surgically or medically.

Surgical evacuation is usually performed under general anaesthetic and the tissue is removed by suction. There is a small risk of uterine perforation, which will need repair.

The medical method is by giving prostaglandin tablets or pessaries, which cause the uterus to contract and expel its contents within 48 hours.

Ectopic pregnancy

Occasionally a pregnancy implants in an 'ectopic' site outside the cavity of the uterus (see page 24). This ectopic site is most commonly in the fallopian tube. The strength of the wall of the tube is insufficient to support the developing embryo and haemorrhage with rupture will eventually occur.

Symptoms of an ectopic pregnancy

The symptoms associated with ectopic pregnancy may be similar to those of miscarriage with bleeding and lower abdominal pain in early pregnancy. If the fallopian tube ruptures, severe pain is experienced, often on one side. If there is excessive bleeding, the patient becomes pale and may faint or collapse completely. With early pregnancy scanning, many ectopic pregnancies are now diagnosed before these severe clinical features develop. The ultrasound scan may show that there is no pregnancy within the uterus. It rarely picks up the actual ectopic pregnancy. The diagnosis is not always easy to make with certainty and the doctor has to be certain that it is not a very early viable intrauterine pregnancy. Sometimes the human chorionic gonadotrophin (hCG) levels need to be checked over a few days to see if the level is rising (the levels normally double every 48 hours in a viable pregnancy).

Treatment

The treatment for an ectopic pregnancy is surgical removal of part or all of the fallopian tube. This is more commonly undertaken by key hole surgery through two or three small (two-centimetre) skin incisions using telescopic instruments (laparoscopic surgery).

Occasionally surgery is not necessary for very small ectopic pregnancies and an injection of the drug called methotrexate can be effective as it causes cellular death in the ectopic pregnancy tissue. After the injection, the hCG levels require monitoring to check that they are falling and that the pregnancy is failing.

Termination of pregnancy because of fetal abnormality

Great sadness will be experienced when a serious abnormality is diagnosed prenatally. Until the abnormality had been found, the baby was considered normal and very much wanted. Choosing to end a pregnancy is a difficult and painful decision. Feelings of guilt and anger are normal and it is important that grieving occurs in whichever way suits the parents. The maternity staff will provide support and guidance. Help groups can be contacted if required (see 'Useful information', page 171).

With the widespread use of ultrasound and invasive testing, serious fetal abnormality can be diagnosed before the stage of viability and so give you the option of termination.

The most common examples of such problems are Down syndrome and spina bifida. The diagnosis of abnormality is usually made in the second three months of pregnancy.

The affected pregnancy is usually terminated by inducing labour. The uterus is first prepared by giving mifepristone by mouth to make the uterus more responsive to prostaglandins. These are then given after 24 to 48 hours in tablet form by mouth or vaginally and they bring on the contractions of labour. The fetus is much smaller at this gestation compared with 40 weeks and so the cervix does not have to dilate so much.

Perinatally related death

Babies still die around the time of birth (perinatally related death) and when this happens it may come as a great shock to parents who have high expectations of modern medicine. It is also difficult for the doctors and midwives – they provide a high standard of care and yet despite all efforts they have failed.

Grief after a perinatal death is extreme. A loved one has gone and there has been very little time with that person. From the excitement of being pregnant and the anticipation of a healthy baby, the opposite emotion of the gloom of death has been reached. Coping with this complicated emotional turmoil is difficult. Feelings of anger, hurt and guilt are not unusual. The maternity hospital staff play a vital role in caring for the bereaved parents and will give help with the registration of death and funeral arrangements. It can be difficult working through the grief reaction and the pain of the loss is never forgotten. For patients having difficulty, support groups may help (see 'Useful information', page 171).

A perinatally related death is one in which there is a pregnancy-associated cause for the death. The deaths are also categorised according to when they occur:

Stillbirth

This is a baby born after 24 weeks of pregnancy who did not breathe or show any other sign of life.

Neonatal death

This is a baby dying within the first four weeks of life regardless of the length of pregnancy. An early neonatal death is one during the first week of life and a late neonatal death is one during the second to fourth week of life.

Postneonatal death

This is a baby dying after four weeks from birth and before the end of the first year.

Infant death

The term 'infant death' refers to any death during the first year of life and will include deaths such as sudden infant death syndrome which are not a result of pregnancy problems.

In 1,000 births about five stillbirths and four neonatal deaths will occur. Another three deaths may occur up to one year after birth. In less developed countries, the death rates may be up to ten times higher. This reflects how better standards of living with improved medical care affect the perinatal mortality rates. Improved nutrition, prevention of disease and education over the last century have been associated with falling perinatal death rates. Factors associated with increased risk are age (under 20, over 35), large number of pregnancies, ethnic minorities and poverty.

In the developed world, significant advances in care have been made, particularly for the pre-term baby. This means that, if the mother has developed complications, such as pre-eclampsia, her baby can be delivered at an earlier gestation than previously. Many babies now survive who would previously have died without modern neonatal care. However, if born at a very early gestation, such as 24 to 27 weeks, they risk developing cerebral palsy as a consequence of the complications of extreme prematurity.

Maternal mortality

Fortunately this is a rare event in industrialised nations but sadly not so in developing countries. The average lifetime risk of death from pregnancy-related causes is 1 in 10,000 maternities whereas in developing countries it is a staggering 1 in 50. The introduction of antibiotics, blood transfusion and better training of midwives and doctors resulted in a dramatic fall in maternal deaths in the 1940s in this country. The introduction of such seemingly simple measures would have a similar effect in developing countries.

In the UK, a report on maternal deaths is issued every three years. All maternal deaths within one year of birth are looked at by an expert panel. Deaths may be directly or indirectly attributable to a pregnancy-related cause. The panel look for any avoidable factors so that lessons may be learned and maternity hospitals advised accordingly.

In the last report suicide was the leading cause overall and advice was given that patients with a history of psychiatric illness should be identified for additional care and support. It was also noted that women in lower social class categories, women from travelling communities, non-white and non-English-speaking women, victims of domestic violence, poor attenders for antenatal care and young women under 18 years of age were all over-represented. Service providers were advised to ensure that the maternity care needs of these disadvantaged women were addressed and met.

KEY POINTS

■ About one in five pregnancies ends in miscarriage

■ In the UK, around 1 in 200 pregnancies ends in stillbirth and 1 in 250 in neonatal death

■ In the UK, the risk of maternal death is 1 in 10,000 pregnancies

Over-the-counter medications

Pregnant women should check with a doctor and/or pharmacist before taking any medicines.

There are some medicines that are considered safe to use in pregnancy and can be purchased from a pharmacy without prescription. However, all medicines should be avoided if possible during the first three months of pregnancy.

Medicine	Purpose
Anusol cream	Apply to soothe haemorrhoids (piles)
Canesten	Vaginal pessary for thrush (*Candida*) and mixed vaginal infections where trichomonas infection may be present
Folic acid	Taken before conception and for the first 12 weeks of pregnancy to reduce the risk of having a fetus with spina bifida
Gaviscon advance	Heartburn
Glycerin suppositories	Constipation
Fybogel	Constipation
Lactulose	Constipation
Maalox/Mucogel	Heartburn/indigestion
Paracetamol	Use for pain caused by backache, headache, symphyseal separation, painful swelling of hands and postnatal perineal pain
Strepsils	Sore throat (see packet)

Useful information

Where can I find out more?

We have included the following organisations because, on preliminary investigation, they may be of use to the reader. However, we do not have first-hand experience of each organisation and so cannot guarantee the organisation's integrity. The reader must therefore exercise his or her own discretion and judgement when making further enquiries.

Active Birth Centre

25 Bickerton Road
London N19 5JT
Tel: 020 7281 6760
Fax: 020 7263 8098
Email: mail@activebirthcentre.com
Website: www.activebirthcentre.com

Offers information, arranges courses and workshops on all aspects of pregnancy and birth. Mail order catalogue including hire of birth pool; details on request.

ARC (Antenatal Results and Choices)

73 Charlotte Street
London W1T 4PN

Tel: 020 7631 0280
Fax: 020 7631 0280
Helpline: 020 7631 0285 (Mon–Fri 10am–5.30pm)
Email: info@arc-uk.org
Website: www.arc-uk.org

Offers information, newsletter and support to parents
through antenatal screening and tests via network of
trained parent contacts.

Association for Postnatal Illness

145 Dawes Road
London SW6 7EB
Tel: 020 7386 0868 (Mon–Wed Fri 10am–2pm, Tues
and Thurs 10am–5pm)
Fax: 020 7386 8885
Email: info@apni.org
Website: www.apni.org

Offers information, advice and support to sufferers of
postnatal illness and their families. Has network of
local contacts.

Benefits Enquiry Line

Tel: 0800 882200
Minicom: 0800 243355
Website: www.dwp.gov.uk
N. Ireland: 0800 220674

Government agency giving information and advice on
sickness and disability benefits for people with
disabilities and their carers.

British Homeopathic Association

Hahnemann House, 29 Park Street West
Luton LU1 3BE
Tel: 0870 444 3950
Fax: 0870 444 3960
Email: info@trusthomeopathy.org
Website: www.trusthomeopathy.org

Professional body offering information about all aspects
of homoeopathy and list of accredited homoeopathic
practitioners in the NHS and private practice.

British Pregnancy Advisory Service (BPAS)

4th Floor, Amec House
Timothy's Bridge Road
Stratford upon Avon CV37 9BF
Tel: 0870 365 5050
Fax: 0870 365 5051
Helpline: 0845 730 4030 (Mon–Fri 8am–9pm; Sat
8.30am–6pm; Sun 9.30am–2.30pm)
Email: comm@bpas.org
Website: www.bpas.org

UK clinics offer pregnancy testing, emergency
contraception and counselling. Book appointments for
terminations of pregnancy, sterilisations and
vasectomies. Translators can be arranged for non-
English speakers.

Citizens Advice Bureaux

Myddelton House, 115–123 Pentonville Road
London N1 9LZ
Tel: 020 7833 2181 (admin only)
Website: www.adviceguide.org.uk

HQ of national charity offering a wide variety of practical, financial and legal advice. Network of local charities throughout the UK listed in phone books and in *Yellow Pages* under 'C'.

Family Planning Association
Floor 2, Featherstone Street
London EC1Y 8QU
Tel: 020 7608 5240
Fax: 0845 123 2349
Helpline: 0845 310 1334 (Mon–Fri 9am–6pm)
Website: www.fpa.org.uk

Offers telephone advice on contraception and sexual health. Appointment needed to view their reference library. Has a useful source of up-to-date information about other services and organisations relating to women's health.

Foresight (Pre-Conceptual Care)
178 Hawthorn Road
West Bognor, W. Sussex PO21 2UY
Tel: 01243 868001
Fax: 01243 868180
Email: min.barnes@foresight-preconception.org.uk
Website: www.foresight-preconception.org.uk

Offers advice about pre-conceptual care and unexplained fertility. For written information, please send an SAE.

Genetic Interest Group
Unit 4D, Leroy House, 436 Essex Road
London N1 3QP
Tel: 020 7704 3141

Fax: 020 7359 1447
Email: mail@gig.org.uk
Website: www.gig.org.uk

Involved in policy-making to protect and improve services, this umbrella organisation represents charities offering support to children, families and individuals affected by genetic disorders.

Gingerbread
(organisation for lone-parent families)

307 Borough High Street
London SE1 1JH
Tel: 020 7403 9500
Fax: 020 7403 9533
Helpline: 0800 018 4318 (Mon–Fri 10am–3pm)
Email: office@gingerbread.org.uk
Website: www.gingerbread.org.uk

National network of self-help groups for lone parents and children. Has publications and advice line covering legal, benefits and emotional issues.

Home-Start

2 Salisbury Road
Leicester LE1 7QR
Tel: 0116 233 9955
Fax: 0116 233 0232
Helpline: 0800 068 6368
Email: info@home-start.org.uk
Website: www.home-start.org.uk

Organisation of trained volunteers, usually parents themselves, operating throughout the UK and British

Forces in Germany and Cyprus. Offers support and practical help in the home to parents with pre-school children in local communities.

Miscarriage Association

c/o Clayton Hospital, Northgate
Wakefield, W. Yorkshire WF1 3JS
Tel: 01924 200795
Fax: 01924 298834
Helpline: 01924 200799 (Mon–Fri 9am–4pm). Also has out of hours message
Email: info@miscarriageassociation.org.uk
Website: www.miscarriageassociation.org.uk
Scottish helpline: 0131 334 8883

Offers information and support by volunteers who have themselves experienced pregnancy loss on miscarriage and ectopic pregnancy. Has UK-wide self-help support groups.

National Childbirth Trust

Alexandra House, Oldham Terrace
London W3 6NH
Tel: 0870 770 3236
Fax: 0870 770 3237
Helpline: 0870 444 8707
Breast-feeding counselling helpline: 08704 448 708 (8am–10pm, 365 days a year)
Email: enquiries@nct.org
Website: www.nctpregnancyandbabycare.com

Parent-to-parent support via local groups. Offers information and pre- and postnatal classes and breast-feeding counselling by trained teachers.

NHS Direct
Tel: 0845 4647 (24 hours, 365 days a year)
Textphone: 0845 606 4647
Website: www.nhsdirect.nhs.uk
NHS Scotland: 0800 224488

Offers confidential health-care advice, information and referral service. A good first port of call for any health advice.

NHS Smoking Helpline
Tel: 0800 169 0169 (7am–11pm, 365 days a year)
Website: www.givingupsmoking.co.uk
Pregnancy smoking helpline: 0800 169 9169 (12 noon–9pm, 365 days a year)
N. Ireland: 0800 858585 (12 noon–11pm, 365 days a year)
Scotland: 0800 848484 (12 noon–12 midnight, 365 days a year)
Wales: 0800 085 2219

Have advice, help and encouragement on giving up smoking. Specialist advisers available to offer ongoing support to those who genuinely are trying to give up smoking. Can refer to local branches.

National Institute for Health and Clinical Excellence (NICE)
MidCity Place, 71 High Holborn
London WC1V 6NA
Tel: 020 7067 5800
Fax: 020 7067 5801
Email: nice@nice.org.uk
Website: www.nice.org.uk

Provides national guidance on the promotion of good health and the prevention and treatment of ill-health. Patient information leaflets are available for each piece of guidance issued.

One Parent Families
255 Kentish Town Road
London NW5 2LX
Tel: 020 7428 5400
Fax: 020 7482 4851
Helpline: 0800 018 5026 (Mon–Fri 9am–5pm and Wed 9am–8pm)
Email: info@oneparentfamilies.org.uk
Website: www.oneparentfamilies.org.uk

Provides free information in 10 languages to lone parents on a variety of issues: maintenance, tax credits, benefits, work, education, legal rights, childcare and holidays.

Parentline Plus
520 Highgate Studios, 53–79 Highgate Road
Kentish Town
London NW5 1TL
Tel: 020 7284 5500
Fax: 020 7284 5501
Helpline: 0808 800 2222 (24 hours)
Textphone: 0800 783 6783
Email: centraloffice@parentlineplus.org.uk
Website: www.parentlineplus.org.uk

Provides general information and runs parenting courses on a variety of issues including bullying, discipline and relationships. Accepts referral via Social Services.

Prodigy Website

Sowerby Centre for Health Informatics at Newcastle
(SCHIN)
Bede House, All Saints Business Centre
Newcastle upon Tyne NE1 2ES
Tel: 0191 243 6100
Fax: 0191 243 6101
Email: prodigy-enquiries@schin.co.uk
Website: www.prodigy.nhs.uk

A website mainly for GPs giving information for
patients listed by disease plus named self-help
organisations.

Quit (Smoking Quitlines)

211 Old Street
London EC1V 9NR
Tel: 020 7251 1551
Fax: 020 7251 1661
Helpline: 0800 002200
Email: info@quit.org.uk
Website: www.quit.org.uk
Scotland: 0800 848484
Wales: 0800 169 0169 (NHS Smoking Helpline)

Offers advice on giving up smoking in English and
Asian languages. Talks to schools on smoking and
pregnancy and can refer to local support groups. Runs
training courses for professionals. Separate helplines
for Scotland and Wales.

Royal College of Obstetricians and Gynaecologists

27 Sussex Place, Regents Park
London NW1 4RG
Tel: 020 7772 6200
Website: www.rcog.org.uk

Provides up-to-date guidelines and information on women's health issues.

SANDS
(Stillbirth and Neonatal Death Society)

28 Portland Place
London W1B 1LY
Tel: 020 7436 7940
Fax: 020 7436 3715
Helpline: 020 7436 5881(Mon–Fri 10am–5pm)
Email: helpline@uk-sands.org
Website: www.uk-sands.org

Offers information and support, via local self-help groups and email, to parents and their families whose babies have died before, during or shortly after birth. Also offers support and training to health-care professionals. Suggests links to many other organisations.

Twins and Multiple Births Association (TAMBA)

The Willows, Gardner Road
Guildford GU1 4PG
Tel: 0870 770 3305
Fax: 0870 770 3303
Helpline: 0800 138 0509 (10am–1pm and 7–10pm, 365 days a year)
Website: www.tamba.org.uk

A parent support organisation that offers training for health and education professionals. Has information leaflets and can refer to local TAMBA groups. Membership brings additional information and support.

Women's Health Concern Ltd

Whitehall House, 41 Whitehall
London SW1A 2BY
Tel: 020 7451 1377
Fax: 020 7925 1505
Helpline: 0845 123 2319
Email: info@womens-health-concern.org
Website: www.womens-health-concern.org

Offers a range of leaflets and fact sheets providing unbiased, accurate information backed by eminent medical advisers.

Working Families

1–3 Berry Street
London EC1V 0AA
Tel: 020 7253 7243
Fax: 020 7253 6253
Helpline: 0800 013 0313
Email: office@workingfamilies.org.uk
Website: www.workingfamilies.org.uk

Works with employers and government on employment-related policies and workplace changes that will benefit families, employers and communities. Offers free advice on employment related issues for working families on legal rights and flexible working hours.

Useful link

Women's Health
www.womenshealthlondon.org.uk

Provides information on gynaecological and sexual health issues.

The internet as a further source of information

After reading this book, you may feel that you would like further information on the subject. The internet is of course an excellent place to look and there are many websites with useful information about medical disorders, related charities and support groups.

For those who do not have a computer at home some bars and cafes offer facilities for accessing the internet. These are listed in the Yellow Pages under 'Internet Bars and Cafes' and 'Internet Providers'. Your local library offers a similar facility and has staff to help you find the information that you need.

It should always be remembered, however, that the internet is unregulated and anyone is free to set up a website and add information to it. Many websites offer impartial advice and information that has been compiled and checked by qualified medical professionals. Some, on the other hand, are run by commercial organisations with the purpose of promoting their own products. Others still are run by pressure groups, some of which will provide carefully assessed and accurate information whereas others may be suggesting medications or treatments that are not supported by the medical and scientific community.

Unless you know the address of the website you

want to visit – for example, www.familydoctor.co.uk – you may find the following guidelines useful when searching the internet for information.

Search engines and other searchable sites

Google (www.google.co.uk) is the most popular search engine used in the UK, followed by Yahoo! (http://uk.yahoo.com) and MSN (www.msn.co.uk). Also popular are the search engines provided by Internet Service Providers such as Tiscali and other sites such as the BBC site (www.bbc.co.uk).

In addition to the search engines that index the whole web, there are also medical sites with search facilities, which act almost like mini-search engines, but cover only medical topics or even a particular area of medicine. Again, it is wise to look at who is responsible for compiling the information offered to ensure that it is impartial and medically accurate. The NHS Direct site (www.nhsdirect.nhs.uk) is an example of a searchable medical site.

Links to many British medical charities can be found at the Association of Medical Research Charities' website (www.amrc.org.uk) and at Charity Choice (www.charitychoice.co.uk).

Search phrases

Be specific when entering a search phrase. Searching for information on 'cancer' will return results for many different types of cancer as well as on cancer in general. You may even find sites offering astrological information. More useful results will be returned by using search phrases such as 'lung cancer' and 'treatments for lung cancer'. Both Google and Yahoo! offer an advanced search option that includes the ability to search for the exact phrase, enclosing the search phrase in quotes, that is, 'treatments for lung cancer' will have the same effect. Limiting a search to an exact phrase reduces the number of results returned but it is best to refine a search to an exact match only if you are not getting useful results with a normal search. Adding 'UK' to your search term will bring up mainly British sites, so a good phrase might be 'lung cancer' UK (don't include UK within the quotes).

Always remember the internet is international and unregulated. It holds a wealth of valuable information but individual sites may be biased, out of date or just plain wrong. Family Doctor Publications accepts no responsibility for the content of links published in this series.

Index

Your pages

We have included the following pages because they may help you manage your illness or condition and its treatment.

Before an appointment with a health professional, it can be useful to write down a short list of questions of things that you do not understand, so that you can make sure that you do not forget anything.

Some of the sections may not be relevant to your circumstances.

We are always pleased to receive constructive criticism or suggestions about how to improve the books. You can contact us at:

Email: familydoctor@btinternet.com
Letter: Family Doctor Publications
         PO Box 4664
         Poole
         BH15 1NN

Thank you

Health-care contact details

Name:

Job title:

Place of work:

Tel:

Name:

Job title:

Place of work:

Tel:

Name:

Job title:

Place of work:

Tel:

Name:

Job title:

Place of work:

Tel:

Significant past health events – illnesses/ operations/investigations/treatments

Event	Month	Year	Age (at time)

Appointments for health care

Name:

Place:

Date:

Time:

Tel:

Name:

Place:

Date:

Time:

Tel:

Name:

Place:

Date:

Time:

Tel:

Name:

Place:

Date:

Time:

Tel:

Appointments for health care

Name:

Place:

Date:

Time:

Tel:

Name:

Place:

Date:

Time:

Tel:

Name:

Place:

Date:

Time:

Tel:

Name:

Place:

Date:

Time:

Tel:

Current medication(s) prescribed by your doctor

Medicine name:

Purpose:

Frequency & dose:

Start date:

End date:

Medicine name:

Purpose:

Frequency & dose:

Start date:

End date:

Medicine name:

Purpose:

Frequency & dose:

Start date:

End date:

Medicine name:

Purpose:

Frequency & dose:

Start date:

End date:

Other medicines/supplements you are taking, not prescribed by your doctor

Medicine/treatment:

Purpose:

Frequency & dose:

Start date:

End date:

Medicine/treatment:

Purpose:

Frequency & dose:

Start date:

End date:

Medicine/treatment:

Purpose:

Frequency & dose:

Start date:

End date:

Medicine/treatment:

Purpose:

Frequency & dose:

Start date:

End date:

Questions to ask at appointments
(Note: do bear in mind that doctors work under great time pressure, so long lists may not be helpful for either of you)

Questions to ask at appointments

(Note: do bear in mind that doctors work under great time
pressure, so long lists may not be helpful for either of you)

Notes